In this book, it is great to see writing from several perspectives that I think will be very useful for parents and professionals alike.
— Garrett Burris, M.D.

I read the book twice and enjoyed it very much. I learned so much about Ryan and the journey his family has experienced; much more than I did in my role as an orthopaedic surgeon. I think this is an important story that needs to be shared. It gives perspectives to physicians, therapists, social workers and legislators who very much need this sort of information and feedback.
— Enrico Stazzone, M.D.

This book is a must read for any family raising a child with special needs. Theresa shares how important a mother's intuition is from the very beginning and that both mothers and fathers have insight that should not be minimized by doctors and other care givers. Theresa's message of hope and perseverance is so heart-felt that it will inspire everyone, especially families caring for those with special needs.
— Heidi Pelant Gioia, WHNP-BC
(Woman's Health Nurse Practitioner, Board Certified)

Dear Ryan, *is an intimate account of a mother's odyssey with her handicapped son through heart-felt letters. Theresa's book is filled with faith in uncertainty, unexpected joys and the bravery of a mother advocating for her child. As a mother, myself, I stand in awe of her strength and honesty. A gem of a book!*
— Amy Inman, Founder-MemoryBox Films and Mother

I was not able to put the book down. It is amazing.
— Maggie Weik, author, Special Needs Adoption
Advocate, and mother of 10

This remarkable and faith-inspiring journey takes us through the gamut of human emotion: The inexplicable bond between a mother and her child, epic challenges, and, ultimately, the ongoing triumph of faith and unconditional love!

— John Wargacki, Associate Professor of English, Seton Hall University

Dear Theresa has given our Dear Ryan a voice that encourages families navigating the difficult but enriching journey with a disabled child from pre-birth expectations to adulthood. Her experiences provide valuable guidance for maximizing a loved one's potential, whatever age or challenges. Theresa shares her story in a non-traditional way demonstrating her strength, wisdom, patience, humor, and a cheerful heart.

— Susan M. Hofmann, P.T.

Enthralled from the first page, I was skillfully led on an emotional journey of a very special boy's influence on so many lives, and then I finished feeling only joy and happiness!

— Brian Mutsch, Lieutenant Commander, U.S. Navy

This book is not just for parents of children with disabilities, it is for all parents. Actually, everyone needs to read this book!

— Patricia Held, mother of five, grandmother of 13, great grandmother and great aunt ("Gigi") to many more.

With brilliant insight, humor and love, Theresa Jeevanjee provides us the moving opportunity to witness the ultimate joy that comes with being the mother of a special needs child. For everyone who has known love, this is the gripping reminder of what makes life truly important. Don't be surprised when you catch yourself binge-reading!

— Nancy Verde, Director of Advising, Fontbonne University

Dear Ryan

Letters, Reflections, and Stories Sharing the
Dance Through Life with a Handicapped Son

By Ryan's Mom,
Theresa Jeevanjee,
Ph.D., C.S.J.A.

Dear Ryan
Letters, Reflections, and Stories Sharing the
Dance Through Life with a Handicapped Son
Theresa Jeevanjee, PhD., C.S.J.A.
FAR Love Press

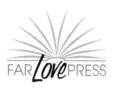

Published by FAR Love Press, St. Louis, MO
Copyright ©2015 Theresa Jeevanjee
All rights reserved.

Editor: Lisbeth Tanz, www.TheHiredPen.com
Proofreader: Karen Garcia, www.TransBloggerForHire.com
Cover and Interior design: Davis Creative, www.daviscreative.com

Library of Congress Cataloging-in-Publication Data
Library of Congress Control Number: 2015905322
Theresa Jeevanjee
Dear Ryan: Letters, Reflections, and Stories Sharing the Dance Through Life with a Handicapped Son
ISBN: 978-0-9961774-0-5
Library of Congress subject headings:
          1. Medical   2. Family and General Practice

2015

Dedicated to:

My husband, Zulfi,
and to our two daughters, Kiran and Lauren.
Thank you for being such wonderful and helpful
companions on this journey with Ryan.

And to all parents everywhere
and those who support them.
I hope sharing our journey
makes yours a little easier.

And, of course, to my dear Ryan,
who from the very beginning,
even before I first held him,
inspired me to write.

Table of Contents

All journal entries, letters and documents from others included in this book are in their raw state and printed as written. I felt it was important to maintain the voice and original writing for authenticity's sake.

1

The Beginning

Let's start at the very beginning;
a very good place to start.
– Earl King Johnson
("Do-Re-Mi" from *The Sound of Music*)

Introduction

I was born in Munich, Germany in 1960, the second child of George Darby, Sr., and Kathleen Logan, who, like most parents, were doing the best they could, especially raising kids while serving in the U.S. Army, which had its own challenges. We had moved 27 times before I was 13. Military life is hard; well, all life can be hard. This book is not about me, but I trust those who said I must tell enough about me for the reader to understand Ryan and my journey with him.

I never thought I would write a book; I write journal articles about mathematics, not books. However, I kept writing stories, letters, and reflections, and, whenever I shared them, nearly everyone kept telling me that I needed to write a book. One of the most enthusiastic and consistent encouragers was my beautiful art teacher, Susan Pisoni. I am grateful to her for encouraging me, and for putting up with me for decades.

This book is for all the people who have walked this journey with us and encouraged me to write about it, believing others would benefit reading about our journey with Ryan. In addition, I am indebted to my early editors (Patricia Held, Sherri Darby, Kenneth Darby, Brian Mutsch, John Wargacki, Jeanne Kloeckner, Nancy Verde, Amy Inman, Maggie Weik) as well as my professional editor, Lisbeth Tanz. I am grateful to Patrick Overton for allowing me to use his poem *Faith* in this book. His poem and faith have been such an important part of my journey.

Throughout this journey with Ryan, I have learned that there is a good deal seriously wrong with the care of people with disabilities. What if my journey could help make that better? I started believing that "they" were right — I needed to write a book. I joined a couple writing groups, checked out some websites, dusted off my pregnancy journal and reflections, and started to believe.

One of the early encouragements was, "If you think you have a story to tell, then you do. Just write it." So, in that spirit, I wrote this book, which is really a collection of many letters, reflections, anecdotes, and stories. It is my hope that it will inspire all parents, not just parents of children (including adult children) with disabilities. In some sense, I suppose we all have "disabilities" or, to use the more politically correct term, "different abilities." Besides, my favorite aunt, who was the very first I trusted with reading the very rough and incomplete draft, said, "It's not just a book for parents of kids with disabilities; it's a book for ALL parents, heck, EVERY-ONE needs to read this." I was humbled and encouraged by her support. I am hopeful that those who choose to read it will get a sense of the sometimes glorious, sometimes arduous journey we are still on with Ryan.

While I do not want this story to be about me, I trust those who have said I should say more about me, and I shall. After all, I suppose I must agree there is no way to tell the story about Ryan without sharing at least some things about me, his mom. After all, I only became the "me" I am now after there was Ryan.

It is also my hope that I do not offend too many folks, but I will say upfront that I am not the most politically correct person on the planet. I think the word offend should be spelled "off-end," because sometimes we all need to be knocked "off" our "ends." While it is rarely my intention to offend anyone, if this book knocks some off their ends, then maybe that is OK. I will leave that up to them.

I am a work in progress, and I encourage folks to read this book as though it comes straight from the heart of an imperfect mother who loves all three of her children. Those who know me well have said that I love ALL children regardless of ability and outward appearance.

I grew up poor in a relatively prosperous America and was a teenager in the 1970s. Ours was the only family I knew who was poor. For us, poor did not mean doing without designer clothes and the latest gadgets, it often meant not having enough to eat and wearing the hand-me-downs of my older brother, George, Jr., to school. Sadly, this was due largely to alcoholism.

Our alcoholic father was in the army, and so we moved a lot —
more than once a year, not including the fifth grade where I got to
spend the whole year in one school. My most vivid memory of childhood was crying myself to sleep the night before starting a new school
— again. It might be hard for folks who know me now to believe, but
I was painfully shy and introverted. Because we moved so much, the
concept of home as a place became incomprehensible to me. Home is
simply where the people I love are, regardless of location.

George and I were and are very close, both in age and in other ways.
While he picked on me a great deal when we were young, he protected
me even more. I used to tease that he made sure no one else beat up on
me so he could. He never hurt me badly and even ran out in the street
once to save me from getting hurt by a car I did not see.

We were all we had for many years. I learned later that our mother had
three miscarriages between having me and our brother, Kenny, and Kenny almost did not make it. I often wish my mother had not died young at
age 48, but I wished it most especially after my third miscarriage.

The divorce of my parents at age 13 seemed almost like a non-event;
although I am sure, it affected me more than it felt at the time. I have
few memories of my father and even fewer good ones. Shortly after
their divorce, Mom remarried a man named Pete, the father of my two
half brothers, Steven and Brian. My mother had to work, and taking
care of the younger children fell to me. So, just as I had taken care of
Kenny, I took care of Steven and Brian. This responsibility made me
grow up fast.

One of my most vivid memories of my mother was of her descriptions of each of us: "George takes after his father, Kenny takes after me,
Steven takes after his father, Brian takes after Teri (my childhood nick-
name) and Teri takes after herself." I never got the chance to ask Mom
before she died what she meant by that. Actually, I am sure I had several
chances, but never did. I wanted it to mean both that I am self-sufficient

and that I do not follow others. Taking after myself (in both senses) and taking care of others are important to me.

One of the few memories I do have of my father was that he bragged that he would pay for me to go to Princeton. Since I was always good in school, I was happy about this and held onto that dream like a touchstone. When I visited him once at age 16, he declared, "Girls do not need to go to college, they just need to get married and have children." Devastated, I realized if I were to go to college, it would be up to me. I do not think I intentionally set out to prove him wrong, but I was well on my way to a Ph.D in mathematics before either of his sons got a bachelor's degree.

After Mom had married Pete, we moved to Niceville, Florida. I lived there for seven years, longer than anywhere else I had ever lived until moving to St. Louis. I finished junior high (now called middle school), high school and junior college all in the same town. I recall often feeling restless. At least once a year I remember thinking, "It must be time to move."

While I excelled in high school, had several honors and the third highest grade point average in a class of 500 students, I had no support from home for college preparation or selection. As a result, I accepted the two-year scholarship to the local junior college that is offered to the valedictorian or salutatorian, who of course never take it because they always have better options. If I knew then what I know now, I would have sought more appropriate options. Back then, I just didn't know better.

After completing my two-year degree, I was lost for a long while. I had developed an eating disorder, was working far too hard and looking for happiness in the wrong places. I found my way back to college at the University of Houston. I finished my bachelor's degree, magna cum laude, in math and computer science just a couple years "late" while working more than full time.

During that time, I met a wonderful man, Emil, who saved my life in many ways. I know he helped me grow a great deal, and I probably should have said yes when he asked me to marry him. I told myself that 13 years was too big of an age gap and talked myself out of marrying him for that and other reasons, none of which I can recall. Looking back, I am sure we would have been happily married, but I would not have Ryan, and so I cannot say I made the wrong choice. There is no doubt in my mind that I was born to be "Ryan's mom."

After graduation, I started working in Austin, Texas. There, I met Ryan's biological father Larry, whose job had transferred him from his hometown of St. Louis. This story is not about Larry and me, but I cannot tell the story about Ryan without telling a little of our story. It is, however, hard for me to tell the story honestly without seeming to be critical of us both. We did and continue to do the best we can. Hindsight has taught me that. We have weathered many difficult relationship issues over the years. Yet, there were and are times when he is the best person for me to talk to. I do not regret anything regarding my relationship with Larry because:

1. I learned to stand up and advocate for myself, which later helped me advocate for Ryan.

2. I have Ryan, and no one except Larry could have made him since he carries the chromosomal abnormality that created our beautiful and unique son.

Larry and I divorced when Ryan was three. Larry is still very involved in Ryan's life. Ryan is very close to my husband, Zulfi. Zulfi and I have two beautiful daughters, Kiran and Lauren. Ryan calls Zulfi "Buddy." For what at the time seemed to be obvious reasons, I did not talk a great deal about Larry and Zulfi in my journals. Larry welcomed my invitation to provide his reflections, and I am indebted to my sister-in-law, Sherri, for saying the words (gently) that made me realize that I should do this. Zulfi just wants to read the book when I have finished. I believe the book is better for Sherri's early suggestions and those of the people who read various drafts and who are acknowledged later.

So there you have it; a snapshot of my early life before Ryan came and saved me. The remainder of this book is all about the person who not only changed my life forever, but who surprises and delights me on a daily basis — Ryan.

I invite the reader to begin this journey where I did ...

2

Dear Ryan ...

Before I formed you in the womb I knew you,
and before you were born I dedicated you, ...
– Jeremiah 1:5
http://www.usccb.org/bible

January 20, 1990

My dear little one,

Today I found out you were a boy. Somehow, it made you even more real to me. I want to hold you and give you all the love I have inside for you.

Sometimes I am afraid that will never happen – I guess because I lost a baby so late in pregnancy last year. Everyone tells me to "think positive," and I am trying. You make it easier by moving around so much.

Feeling you move inside me is the most incredible thing I have ever experienced. It's hard to explain, but when I feel you or look down and see my belly move, I am in awe knowing there is another person inside me. A person – someone I will love always. Someone I will try to give my very best. Someone I hope will be happy in this life and Beyond.

Life is hard. Marriage is impossible.

This used to be my mantra. Reading it now makes my throat close. I want to scream. How and when did life become so hard? When did I lose my ability to be happy no matter what?

I did not always think that life was hard, even when it was. In fact, I was usually known as "Smiley" because I was so happy, no matter what. I did not really want much out of life. I did not have any lofty expectations. I did want to be married. I didn't want the kind of marriages my parents experienced, nor did I want to ever get divorced. I was hopeful and believed that being happily married was possible. I did not know anyone who was happily married, but, hey, The Bible talked about it, so surely it was possible.

Later, much later, I experienced a marriage that was not impossible. Much later, my mantra became "Life is Good." But the journey there is the stuff of this book. This is my nonlinear path from an innocent, spiritual seeker to a lost person whose life's goal was to "come down from the mountain." Well, I came down from the mountain and fell face first on the ground with my limbs spread out, exhausted. It was Ryan who led me.

After losing a pregnancy at 18 weeks the year before, I took Clomid to correct a perceived fertility imbalance. It worked the first time I used it. I never thought to question my miscarriage, nor did I know that Clomid rarely works the first time.

Today, I know through research that the child I lost had a chromosomal abnormality related to the one that Ryan has but was unable to remain viable. These extremely rare chromosome disorders are surrounded by wonder and mystery, just like Ryan. I invite the interested reader to check the glossary at the end of the book for more information on chromosomes and for any other acronyms that are not explained.

Miracles

I spent more than half of my life not believing in miracles. I have a mathematical and scientific mind. I believed, actually thought that I knew, that "miracles" were just things that had not yet been explained or simply could not be explained in certain situations. I believed that someday they would be explained, and I do still think that might be true. God does not break the laws of physics and mathematics. Doing that would completely go against my understanding of a loving God who created an organized (for the most part) universe with humans who have free will. This free will ensures the possibility for true happiness and allows for sadness and occasional chaos. No miracles, just unexplained goodness.

I wish I could tell you exactly when I started acknowledging miracles because it would seem that it would have been a big turning point in my life. Notice I used "acknowledging" rather than "believing" because our belief in something is independent of its truth or existence. That I do know.

I suppose it does not matter exactly when I started accepting miracles, but it is important that I somehow went from not believing in miracles to counting on them.

The miracles were always there, and they continued throughout my unbelief. Ryan is a miracle, as are all children, and as is all life. There have been many miracles along our journey.

Another important lesson I learned about miracles is that they remain miracles even when we understand why they occur. For example, understanding the physics behind a rainbow does not take away the miracle of rainbows; in fact, it enhances their beauty – at least for me.

Miracles are essential. I also know that now.

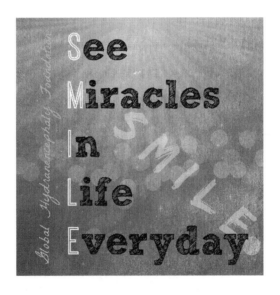

January 25, 1990

Dear Ryan,

Today we went to hear about all the anesthetics available at delivery. It was scary for me because I don't want to do anything to hurt you. I would rather "suffer a natural delivery" than put you in danger. I guess we'll put this in God's hands and pray for strength.

Love,

Your mom

Working it Out

I was worried about anesthetics. I never drank alcohol, diet sodas, or even caffeine while I was pregnant with Ryan. I do not regret doing without any of those things; I only wish being healthy during my pregnancy had ensured his health.

The fact was that no matter what I did, Ryan was still going to be born with severe disabilities. Contemplating this brings to mind the Big Question of Purpose. In the early days, when my life and sanity were hanging on by a thin thread, and someone would say, "Everything happens for a reason," I wanted to strangle them. I am not a violent person. Instead of acting out my initial reaction, I just bit my tongue, sometimes quite literally.

Today, I still have people say to me, "God has a reason for everything, and God is in control." I struggle with this thinking. While I strongly believe that God *could be* in control, it is very hard to accept that God chooses to be in control for several reasons. To accept that God is in control means that God is fixing some things and ignoring others.

That does not work with my idea of a good, loving, and gracious God. I can live with the idea that God gives us freedom so that we can truly love and make order out of the chaos that we sometimes inadvertently create. If God controls us, we are not free to love. If God allows us to be free, then we are free to love, but also free to hate and make bad choices. Our bad choices can infringe on others. What a mess, but that is Life. God is there to help us clean up the mess if we allow God to do that. God *makes* meaning and reason out of everything.

As a professor of mathematics and computer science, I often teach classes in mathematical logic. I sometimes challenge my students with the "paradox" of three seemingly mutually exclusive propositions:
1. God is Good.
2. God is All Powerful.
3. There is Evil in the world.
It seems clear that one of these has to go. However, C.S. Lewis reconciled this paradox in his wonderful book *Mere Christianity*. The propositions are mutually exclusive *if and only if* you assume that "all powerful" means control. God can be all-powerful, but choose not to control. Giving us freedom allows us to love freely. Being free allows freedom of choice. Freedom of choice allows bad choices and even evil as well. It is messy but necessary for true happiness, so ultimately Good. This resolution makes sense to me. It is the foundation upon which I base my life.

January 26, 1990

Dear Ryan,

It is hard to be pregnant. I know it is something you will never experience directly, but I wanted to write down some of my thoughts and experiences to share with you someday.

I started so late because I was afraid to become too attached in case I lost you, which is silly of course, because I became attached immediately.

So, I will try to backtrack and write down some special dates and events in your development while inside of me. ☺

I cried when I found out for certain on August 4, 1989, that I was pregnant with you. I was scared to be pregnant because I had a very late miscarriage last year. I was afraid to love you and then go through the pain of losing you. Your father and I were also struggling in our marriage, and selfishly I thought of all the *things that would now have to wait: graduate school, Europe, Israel. I was also thinking of 9+ months of being sick, tired and fat.*

It did not take long, however, for me to become happy about you and glad that you were a part of me. Having a baby is the neatest experience in the world.

I wonder what you will be like, who you will look like, when you will come. I know I will love you no matter what – forever.

Things We Hold Deep Inside

When I asked Larry, Ryan's father, to contribute his memories to this book, without hesitation, the first thing he recalled was that I cried when I found out I was pregnant. I was surprised that was the first event he remembered. He was worried that I cried because I was not happy to be pregnant. I wish that he had asked me. It might have brought him some comfort to know that my tears were out of fear of *losing* this new life inside of me, not of *having* it.

January 27, 1990

We told your grandparents about you on October 8 by playing your heartbeat for them. They were very excited and also very excited when I told them last week you are a boy. There are many people here waiting to give you lots of love.

I must admit to being a little scared, though. This is a crazy world, and I shudder to think of the harm that could come to you. I usually try to think of all the good in the world, but I have never been responsible for another human being before.

We live in St. Louis, which is a nice place for you to grow. We live in a residential area close to a nice park. I am anxious to take you for walks there and, later, to play on the swings.

If you come on time, it will only be 10 more weeks before I get to hold you!

×later×

Today we bought you a crib, a cradle, a dresser/changing table, and a high chair. Your room is all ready. I hope you like it. I also got a baby-blue Care Bear crib set for you – it is very cute. Your whole room is filled with bears.

What is in a Name?

Picking a name for a child seems to be such a huge task. It will be how people see that child for the rest of his or her life. No pressure!

Larry's family had a tradition of using the names Edward and Lawrence. Larry's father was "Edward Lawrence" and Larry was "Lawrence Edward." I'm not sure why, but we didn't feel that Edward was the right name for our new baby.

We thought Christopher would be a nice name, but I worked with someone named Christopher who was arrogant and egotistical. Unfortunately, he ruined the name for me, at least at that point in my life.

I have always liked the name Ryan, which means "little king" in Gaelic. Since Lawrence means "crowned one," it seemed like a wonderful complement to his family's tradition. Since we are Irish, Ryan seemed perfect. It has been the perfect name. He is a little king, crowned with all of God's goodness. I find it funny that most people call him "Mr. Ryan." And, although Ryan was originally a Gaelic surname, somehow I do not think that is why folks call him Mister.

January 29, 1990

I love you so much, but I'm so scared. I hope I will be a good mom. I want the very best for you.

I have made so many mistakes in my life – I don't want to make any with you. Please, God, help me to be a good mommy.

January 30, 1990

Hi, sweetheart,

Everyone keeps telling me that I am so thin to be 7 months pregnant. Sometimes I get tired of hearing it. I don't feel thin. I have gained over 30 pounds, and I still have 10 weeks to go! I don't mind gaining the weight because I know I am eating right so that you'll be the best I can "make" you.

I want to stay healthy for many reasons – you are one. You deserve to have a mommy who will live as long as possible and be healthy enough to take you on walks and play without getting tired.

I am still running about 5 miles a day. That amazes everyone, too. But I have been doing it for 11 years, and I love it. My runs are more like slow jogs or very fast walks, but they help keep me fit and preserve my sanity.

Today while I was running I got lost in a sort of daydream. I pictured you about 4 years old in Africa with me and a very good friend of mine, Zulfi. He is from Nairobi and he was showing you all the animals. You and I had a long talk in his father's garden. You were asking me all about flowers and a zillion other things.

I think like that a lot. I picture you at different ages and in different situations. I wonder if you'll be like the little boy I picture.

I'm sure you will be full of questions, and I'm sure I will love you no matter what you're like. I pray I have the wisdom and patience to answer all your questions.

You are moving so much these days – sometimes I think you are trying to get out! I love it when you move – it's the best experience a woman can have. I can't even begin to adequately describe the emotion I have when I feel you and when I look *down to see my tummy taking on strange shapes. Keep it up! I love feeling you – it means you are alive and well.*

Mommy

Ryan Came and Saved Me

I think that is a phrase in a song by Sinead O'Connor that I used to play for Ryan. It was also the answer I recently gave to someone who was on our parish's ACTS retreat who seemed to feel very bad for me that I "have a son who is disabled." I did not even take a moment to think about it, "Ryan saved me." She replied, "Everyone I know who has kids with disabilities says that."

For me, the "saving" was early and often. From the beginning, Ryan's existence was responsible for my turning from a path that would likely have ended in death. That may sound dramatic, but it's not meant to be. I firmly believe Ryan came from God to save me and give me the chance to be his mom.

I have not shared with many people that I struggled with anorexia and bulimia, although I am sure that many people suspected it. At 5'8" and between 110 and 115 pounds, I was *far* too skinny. I set out on a path to healthy eating and a healthier weight, the moment I learned I was pregnant with Ryan. I could do for him what I could not do for myself.

February 1, 1990
My Dear Little One,

I love to watch and feel you move. I remember when we first heard your heart beating and first saw you on the ultrasound on October 6. I still have the tape of your heartbeat and the picture of the ultrasound. Someday I will give them to you.

You are kicking like crazy right now – it's hard to write when the book keeps moving. ☺
I love you!
Mom

The first "picture" of Ryan

I recall when we saw the ultrasound. This was long before ultrasounds were as good as they are now. It was amazing to see the image of Ryan inside me. Before we had even decided whether we wanted to know the gender, the technician got a view of "baseball equipment" (balls and bat) so, we knew I was carrying a boy. I was both happy and sad. It was the beginning of a journey of gift and loss. Accepting the gift of one thing means the loss of something else is a valuable lesson that I have not yet fully embraced.

February 2, 1990

Dear Ryan,

Today is Ground Hog's Day, and considering it's so yucky outside, I'm sure we'll have 6 more weeks of winter. That's OK – it hasn't seemed very cold to me since I've been pregnant. And in 9 weeks when you're born, it will be springtime, no matter what the weather.

I'm waiting for the doctor right now. Just a routine check up, but I'll get to hear your heart beat again. Boom, boom, boom – I wish people did not overuse the word awesome. It should be saved for times like these.

Groundhog Day

These many years later, I learned that Groundhog Day was originally all tied up with the feast of the Presentation of Jesus. Seems fitting that we took this picture on that day.

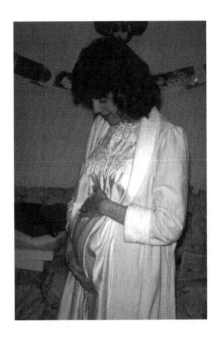

Further Reflection on Groundhog Day

February 2, 2013

Dear Ryan,

As I look at that picture, I recall that as a "Southern Transplant," I was usually cold from October to April in St. Louis. Your paternal grandmother gave me the lovely gown that I am wearing in the picture and your dad gave me the pretty robe to keep me warm. Being pregnant with you was probably the first time during winter that I was not always so cold.

Someone sent me a funny picture yesterday of a wolf who looked upset. The caption was "The groundhog said there would be six more weeks of winter." Down below it added, "So, I ate him." That made us all smile, but because of you, I no longer dislike winter. In fact, I welcome the change of seasons. I love life, no matter what the weather. I even like groundhogs – we had a recent critter situation in the basement, I will tell you about that later.

I love you.

Mommy (who is warm)

February 6, 1990

My precious boy,

Last night I could hardly walk and today is not much better. My pelvic bones hurt so much – I wonder if you are turning over. I hope so.

You have been moving so much lately and I smile every time you do. I love you so much, little one, I hope everything goes well until you're born and after – ever after.

Your mommy

February 7, 1990

Dear Ryan,

I see children EVERYWHERE. I look at their cute little faces and wonder what you will look like. The world seems full of children since I have been pregnant.

I no longer think of the things I will miss by having a baby. I think of the wonderful times I will have with you. The postponement of graduate school; Europe and/or Israel; the decision of whether or not to continue working; the changing of our lifestyles – all seem small now compared with the joys I will experience by having you! I can't wait!

Your mommy

February 8, 1990

My dearest little one,

Tonight we had our first childbirth class. Our instructor is wonderful! She is funny and warm. She is also pregnant, so she is living through it, too. I learned some interesting things. We saw a poster of the inside of a female – no wonder I have to go to the bathroom all the time! The uterus is resting right on the bladder and everything is squished.

It was neat hearing from other moms-to-be what their experiences are; it's nice to know I'm not alone. Of course, I am not alone with you inside me.

I think everything's going to be OK.

I love you.

Mommy

p.s. We went down the hall to the nursery – it's amazing you will be in there soon!

Nursery?

A nursery is a room set apart for small children. My paternal grandmother, Grandma Darby, was a nurse. She actually had a BSN (Bachelor of Science in Nursing) during a time when not many women achieved that, choosing instead for the shorter program in nursing so they could help with the war.

Grandma Darby has long passed but remains in my mind as one of the smartest people I have ever known. She did a great deal to build up my high opinion of nurses. My journey with Ryan has also given us the opportunity to be on the caring end of many good nurses. I bring up nurses here to explain why "nursery" has such a sweet connotation in my mind. A nursery is a place where smart, loving women take care of babies and children.

The nursery in our hospital was not like the image in my mind, although our nurses were all very good. This hospital is known in St. Louis as "the baby factory." This is not necessarily a bad thing; rather it speaks more to the sheer numbers of babies they deliver each year. This alone took away from my image of a quiet, peaceful nursery.

When I close my eyes, I can still see the rows of babies—literally rows of them. They were bundled up in swaddling with beanies on their heads. Some were blue, most were pink. They were all asleep. I am not sure how they managed to sleep in such a loud, bustling environment that was also sterile and cold. I understand the reasons for all of it, but it was not the image of the nursery I had in my mind.

Because the hospital's nursery reality didn't correspond with the mental image I envisioned for Ryan, I decided to do something I rarely did. I asked for something different. "Could I have my son in my room?" I had planned to nurse Ryan, and I thought it would be easier and better to have him close by. My voice was small, but it sounded so loud in my ears because I had yet to become the strong advocate I would later learn that I needed to be for Ryan.

To my happy surprise, the answer was yes. This was true, at least in theory. If there were complications, then the answer would be no.

February 10, 1990

Dear Ryan,

Yesterday was a tough day. You have not been letting me sleep lately, and being tired dampens everything.

I went with my friend, Heidi, to her bi-weekly fetal monitoring test. Yesterday was the same day last year in her pregnancy that she delivered her stillborn baby, Maria. She started having mild contractions in the office, and the doctor wants her on complete bed rest for at least 5 weeks.

I am so sad for her. It is hard enough to be pregnant, especially when you've lost one, without having to lie in bed and think about it. I hope she is OK. I hope YOU are OK.

It doesn't seem fair that there are so many women who have abortions, who abuse their children, even murder them, when there are women like my friends Heidi, Jennifer and like myself who want children so much and have so much trouble having them.

Life is not always fair, Ryan. Sometimes it is cruel in its injustice. But, sometimes it is fair, and sometimes it is wonderful. I hope that in your life the good times outnumber the bad times. They have in mine.

The joy you have already brought me far outweighs the pain and fear.

Love always, Mommy

February 14, 1990

My sweet baby,

Today is Valentine's Day. Your father gave me a card from you signed, "Thanks for having me. Your son, Ryan." I hope you do feel happy someday that we made you.

Mommy

Valentine's Day

I hate Valentine's Day. I believe it to be a contrived holiday to benefit chocolate makers, florists, restaurants, and jewelers. We, especially women, are brought up to expect certain things. I know for many, many years I bought into this. I thought that if I did not get a tangible sign of affection on Valentine's Day, I was not loved or appreciated.

I loved this little note from "Ryan" that Larry wrote. In fact, I still have it. I have always appreciated these kinds of gifts the most. Somehow, when everyone at work got flowers on Valentine's Day, and I did not, I would still feel bad. If the day came and went and no one even called, I felt unloved. I have finally evolved past this. Now, I make reservations for Zulfi and me at my favorite restaurant. It relieves the stress of him having to make plans (not his thing even when he is not busy at work), and I get to do something I enjoy.

Even though I have finally learned to have few expectations on Valentine's Day, I still could live without it.

February 16, 1990

My dear little one,

I think you turned over last night because my tummy was twisting and turning in all directions. I hope that means you are getting in the "right" position. I want very much to deliver you normally.

Most of the time I feel like nothing in my life has ever been normal. I want everything to go right for you from the very beginning.

Our "baby classes" are very interesting and fun. I am less afraid the more I learn in the class or by reading. I am getting so anxious to meet you!!!

Normal

In mathematics, "normal" is a word that can mean different things depending on the context. It can mean everything from canonical (standard) to perpendicular.

In life, it is often hard to determine what "normal" is. It seems popular now to respond with, "What is normal anyway?" whenever someone uses the word. What *is* normal?

Most of the time, I think it is easier to define normal by saying what it is not. It is not normal to do this. It is not normal to do that.

In my early letters to Ryan, I often expressed that I wanted him to be normal. How very un-evolved of me! I am so very glad that God had other plans.

February 24, 1990

Dear baby,

Thursday in childbirth class, we saw a film of labor and delivery – it was neat to see, but scary. I hope that all the pain will result in a healthy you – then it would be well worth it.

Today I changed the ribbons on your baptismal gown from pink to blue. My mom started crocheting this beautiful gown before she died and my favorite aunt finished it as a surprise. So, it is doubly special. Aunt Trish put pink ribbons on it because we all thought the baby I lost before you was a girl.

It's hard to believe you will be here in 6 weeks!!! I can't wait. Please don't strangle yourself on your cord.

Mom

March 4, 1990

My dear little one,

It has been a while since I have written – things have been very busy. Your grandma is in the hospital and I have been very busy at work. My boss is leaving, which means I have more to do and learn. You just moved – I'm so glad you are OK. ☺

Friday the doctor said you are almost in the right position. I was so happy to hear that because I want you to be born naturally.

Today we met another couple who just had a baby. We were at this family's house to "learn" about baptism. It was a very nice afternoon. We saw a film on baptism and then visited with the other couples. I held their 6-week old little girl and tried to imagine what it would be like to hold you. I can't wait.

Mommy

March 7, 1990

Dear Ryan,

Yesterday your godmother took me shopping for baby things. She had a bag full of things for you when I got there and bought you more while we were out. She is excited to meet you, too! I bought a bunch of things, too. I think we're almost ready as far as clothes and things. I've been ready for a long time to meet you.

It was fun being out with Carol and two of her daughters, but it was a little hard, too. I still sometimes worry that something will happen and it will have been foolish for me to get all this stuff. I want so much to hold you and love you.

Mommy

p.s. I hope you like bears. ☺

March 15, 1990

My dear baby,

It's been a while since I have written. I have been so busy at work and tired all the time. You keep me awake most nights.

My friend, Heidi is really having a tough time. Even though she is only 34 weeks pregnant, they will probably let her deliver soon. Her baby will likely only weigh 4 1/2 pounds.

Tonight was our last "baby class." The film we saw about childcare and new parenting was scary. It almost took all the joy out of looking forward to you. All the parents talked about was being tired, no sex, crying babies, etc. etc. I hope it is better for us.

It was a good class, though, and we learned a lot.

Two couples in the class had their babies yesterday. One couple had twins. Seeing them was reassuring – they were so happy.

One girl in the class lost her baby at 8 months. I cried – I feel so bad for her. I don't know if I could take it if anything happens to you.

Something's Wrong

I realized, after reading these two journal entries several times, that I had a premonition that something would be "wrong" with Ryan; it was especially strong on March 15. It was as though God was trying to prepare me. Of course, nothing can truly prepare us for the journey of parenthood, much less the journey we have had.

March 16, 1990

My dear little one,

Today during my exam, the doctor felt your head! That was exciting for me.

I lost a pound and my belly only grew 1 cm, so he was a little concerned. He said it could be because you were in position or because I am thin and long-waisted.

He said he didn't want to jinx things, but judging from things, you would come on time or early. That means three weeks or less!!! I can't wait.

Today I packed some of your things in my suitcase. That was a big statement of Faith on my part that I believe you really are coming. Your things look so small next to mine. But, they Belong there. ☺

March 17, 1990
Dear Ryan,

I am at a cafeteria in the mall taking a break from shopping. It is hard to believe that before long I won't be doing things like this alone any more. You will be with me wherever I go. Different from the way you are with me now, that is. Right now you are a part of me quite literally, wiggling and squirming inside of me. Someday very soon, you will be your own person with your own ideas and dreams.

I want that for you, but at the same time, I don't want to ever let go of you.

Love,

Mommy

p.s. Happy St. Patrick's Day, my Irish son.

Letting Go
April 10, 2014
Dear Ryan,

Reflecting on this again while we are preparing to let your sister, Kiran, go off to college, and prepare your sister, Lauren, for driving, has made me realize that I have gotten to have you at home and hold onto you in ways that I would not have been able to had you been "normal." Part of this journey has been learning to experience the deep joys along with the deep sorrows.

I have learned a great deal about letting go while holding your hand. The following poem has helped lead me...

Faith

When we walk to the edge of all the light we have
and take that step into the darkness of the unknown,
we must believe that one of two things will happen—

There will be something solid for us to stand on
Or, we will be taught how to fly.

– Patrick Overton, "The Leaning Tree" © 1975

March 21, 1990

Dear Ryan,

Your feet are in your favorite spot in my ribs again. I am so ready for you to come! I want to hold you and love you, but, selfishly, I want to feel normal again, too. It has been so long, I'm not sure I know what normal is anymore. ☺

March 22, 1990

My dear little one,

We just witnessed a teenage boy pull his car out in front of another car in front of us, get hit and slide off into a ditch. Fortunately, everyone is okay. We came very close to hitting him ourselves. I shudder to think I could have lost you or someone else could have been hurt because of his foolish hurriedness.

It made me realize that my worries have just begun. I will have concern for you and what others do to you for the rest of my life because I love you so much.

I hope I do not smother you with my love and care.

Mommy

p.s. Please move your foot. It hurts.

March 25, 1990

Dear Ryan,

Today I went to a surprise shower. Daddy's cousin Laura gave it. She told me the shower was for her sister who is due May 1 and that we were supposed to bring a dish to be frozen for her when she comes home from the hospital. What a surprise – the shower was for us! Laura made lots of yummy food and we got lots of very nice things for you. Everyone is so excited for you to come. ESPECIALLY ME!

I just got a call from a running friend who is doing an article for the St. Louis Track Club on pregnant runners. That was neat having someone who was interested in running rather than telling me I should not do it. We had a nice run today, in fact.

I love you so very much. I wish you'd find a different place for your feet, though! ☺

Mommy with bruised ribs.

March 28, 1990

My dear little one,

I am home alone – it's so peaceful and quiet. This is probably the last time for a very long time that it will be this way. You have the hiccups again right now. That is such a funny feeling.

I hope you are ok. I hear so many stories about abnormal babies – it's scary. Only 10 more days till your due date! I love you.

Mommie

Abnormal

My mother made me take Latin in high school. I did not like it at the time. However, it has helped me a great deal, especially with English and

French vocabulary. There are so many words and prefixes that "come for free." *Ab* means "out of." Out of the norm. I reflected earlier that we often understand normal by discovering what something is *not* – how "ab" from normal it is.

Ryan is far from normal, by anyone's definition, and while it has been scary at times, it has been so wonderful. He is the happiest person I know, and I submit with deep gratitude that I am the second happiest. I really no longer believe there is such a thing as normal. And if there is, I want no part of it.

April 1, 1990

My dear little one,

Please do not come today. I do not want your birthday to be April Fool's Day. ☺

You're still moving a great deal. I will never forget the first flutters I felt and the first time you moved and it was visible from the outside. That was November 18, 1989.

You are due next Sunday! I can't wait!!!

Love, Your mom

Reading this many years later, I have to appreciate the diversity that the customs and cultures of different countries bring. And how minor things such as being born on April 1st are in the scheme of things.

St. Louis is fortunate to have a large community of Bosnians who came because of the war and turmoil in their region. We were fortunate to have friends from there, Iris and Sinisa. Iris's birthday is April 1. She of course thought nothing of it until she came to America. I am hopeful that America has solved more problems than it brought. But these minor, funny coincidences have helped me put the fear of your being born on April 1st in perspective. How silly I was in those days.

April 5, 1990

Dear Ryan,

Monday night I had pain and light contractions all night until 6 am. What an exhausting night. I worked Tuesday, but decided that would be my last day. I will log in from home until you are born and probably from now on.

Yesterday was a nice spring day and even more enjoyable because I didn't have to go to work and I got a little sleep.

I am waiting to have a pre-natal conference with your pediatrician, Dr. Marsha (not her real name), and then on to what I hope will be my last OB/Gyn visit before you are born.

I wonder when you will be born. Soon, I hope.

Love, Mommy

April 8, 1990

My dear little one,

Today is your due date, but somehow I was not surprised when the day came and went without any sign of you. I do hope you come soon.

My friend, Heidi, had her baby April 6. She was two and a half weeks early, but that is much better than the ten weeks early she would have been had she delivered back when she first started having contractions. He was 6 lbs. 2 oz., which is great considering his parents are fairly small and that he was early.

I had a nice run today – it was so pretty outside. I got some funny looks, though. Everyone thinks pregnant women shouldn't run.

I still have trouble sometimes believing in you. I must be trying to prepare myself for some unknown disaster. I want so much for you to be normal and healthy *and to be delivered normally.*

I saw a lady in the craft store today who had a son with Down's syndrome. I got the oddest feeling when I looked at this blond little boy. It was as though God was trying to tell me something through him.

I may be selfish, but I pray you have nothing like Down's. I get really scared sometimes. Please come soon; I want to hold you.

Love, Mommy

Wrong, again

This was the day when I knew beyond a shadow of a doubt that something was "wrong" with Ryan. It was one of those life-altering moments you only have to shut your eyes to recall fully – you can see, hear, and feel everything as though it is happening again.

I felt that God had prepared me for this moment my entire life. It is like the stories people tell of their lives "flashing before them" when they taste death but do not meet it. When you look back, you realize it was a defining moment – similar to the memories people have of their whereabouts when major events occurred, such as President Kennedy's death, the Challenger explosion, or the destruction of the Twin Towers. This was the first of several such moments for me. My life to that point "flashed" before me. I remembered Mom taking me with her when she volunteered with mentally retarded children, my independent study involving autistic children that, by a bizarre turn of events, became necessary for my graduation, my volunteering with mentally retarded adults, and countless other moments with "special" children and adults. I also was told I was a "natural" while studying genetics in high school and college. Genetics was a new field, yet I had no trouble grasping the science behind the concepts. It all came easily. On this day, it suddenly felt as if my life had been one big Preparation. I just knew.

The night before Ryan's birth, I could not sleep. I do not suppose that is unusual even in "normal" pregnancies. I finally got out of bed, and, not wanting to wake Larry, called my good friend, Zulfi. I knew he would be awake studying; I tried to tell him what I was feeling. While he tried to be supportive and reassuring at the time, later I would learn that he shared the same fears. This was not the last time Zulfi and I experienced a common foreboding.

April 10, 1990

My dear little one,

This morning we had our "non-stress" test, the one where they monitor movement, heart rate, and contractions. You did fine; I passed out. Once the nurse got you moving, you wouldn't quit!

It looks like tomorrow could be your birthday. We are supposed to be at the hospital by 6:30 am so they can induce labor. I am ready, but scared. I hope we are doing the right thing. Maybe you'll come on your own tonight.

I love you. Mom

Good Friends

The morning I was to be induced, my good friend, Jennifer, met us at the hospital to wish us the best. She has been such a good and faithful friend. She was my first friend when I came to St. Louis in 1987 and remains one of my best friends ever.

There have been many times over the years when "Aunt Jenny" came to the hospital to visit and/or to help us. One time, in particular, stands out when she brought Ryan a change of clothes to St. Luke's — I had put that out of my memory.

April 11/12, 1990

[The writing up to now has been very neat. This entry is wobbly and messy with cross outs. The Demoral had a lot to do with this, I think. ☺]

Dear Ryan,

Last night at 7:28 you were born! We got to the hospital at 6:30 am, but had to wait for a room. [Why does this sound so funny???]

They took us to labor and delivery about 9 am and started the "drip" for inducing labor at 10:30. Labor didn't start until 1 pm and got really painful between 5 and 7 pm when they put in the IV for pain. They had to do an emergency C-section because your heart stopped beating.

This is so sloppy because of the shot they gave me for the incision – it makes me drowsy.

There are no words to describe how I felt when I held you in my arms and touched your soft skin.

More later, Mom

So Soft

I recalled re-reading the above passage that Ryan was so soft that I felt that I was hurting him with my touch. Surely, my hands must have felt like sandpaper to such soft skin. Even today, Ryan still has the softest skin. I'm told my skin is very soft, too, so I suppose that is one trait Ryan got from me.

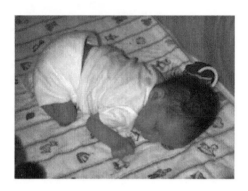

April 13, 1990

Ryan,

We got a real scare when the pediatrician told us there were several things 'not quite right' about you (extra bone on scalp, small soft spot, extra fold on ears, eyes far apart, pointy nose, left testicle not dropped.) She said any one by itself would not have bothered her, but that many caused concern. She ordered a skull x-ray and a chromosome test. The chromosome test results will be ready Monday. What a long time to wait! We are very upset and discouraged.

She called at 7 pm yesterday to tell us the skull x-rays are fine!!! That eliminates lots of things and makes it easier to wait until Monday.

To Cut or Not to Cut

While we waited for test results, we still had to consider Ryan's circumcision. When our OB/Gyn doctor, Dr. S, asked us if we wanted to circumcise Ryan, Larry and I were unsure of what to say. Dr. S promised that he did each one as though he were doing it to himself. He did not believe the common notion that babies do not feel pain. I trusted him.

As usual, I asked for the advantages and disadvantages. It seemed a good thing to do, given that there was less of a risk of infection with circumcision; and there did not seem to be a downside since most Christian American males had it done. I did not really think much about it. I certainly was not projecting into the future or wondering about future relationships for him. I simply could not see that far. I did hope.

April 14, 1990

My Dear Child,

I do not know where to begin. I have reached pinnacles of emotion in all directions. We are still not 'out of the woods' yet with you, and we discovered yesterday that you have a slight heart murmur, which indicates a VSD (a hole in the wall between the ventricular sections of your heart. VSD = ventricular septal defect). It will either close by itself or can be closed by a simple heart surgery, but it was just one more hump in this roller coaster ride that has been the first week of your life. We wanted so much for you to be healthy. I guess we will know for sure on Monday. You also have a touch of jaundice, so they have you under bili lights. It breaks my heart to see you cry!

Nursing you is one of the most beautiful experiences of my life. You seem to know my voice, my touch, and my face. You now open your mouth when they bring you to me. You almost always get quiet when I hold you. We are Connected.

I made a deal with God

As I re-read the entry from April 14, the day we brought Ryan home, "pinnacles of emotions in all directions," does not even begin to describe it. What happened that evening was pivotal for me. I am not sure why I did not write in my "Dear Ryan" journal. Perhaps I thought it was wrong or that I only wanted to share upbeat, positive things in case Ryan ever read it.

My Aunt Patricia (affectionately called Gigi by all her grandchildren and great-grandchildren) came to help us with Ryan when he came home from the hospital. She is a wonderful woman and my mom's younger sister. Aunt Patricia, whom I call Aunt Mom or Aunt Trisha, became a second mother to me after my mom died much too young. After putting Ryan to bed, I went to my bedroom to rest. Larry and Gigi stayed downstairs.

I crawled into the bed so exhausted and very sore from the C-section. I wanted so badly to have Ryan "normally." A reminder of the C-section was now some indeterminate number of staples across my once flat stomach. A C-section was not what I wanted, but became necessary when Ryan's heart stopped. For me, it was the start of signs that I was no longer in control — if I ever was. Zulfi told me once in his lovely British accent, "Control is a Western myth." This was one of the first of many lessons I would learn because of Ryan.

As I lay there, I felt as if I was melting under the covers. It was April and cool, but I was hot. As I shut my eyes, a flashback to the night a year before when I miscarried came unbidden. I had never seen so much blood; our queen-sized bed was covered in it. I was literally gushing blood, as I lost that late-term pregnancy. I later learned that this pregnancy was likely lost due to the monosomy manifestation of Larry's balanced translocation. On this night, while Ryan was sleeping in his bed for the first time, I sobbed for the child I lost, the child I received, and for Ryan's "loss."

Suddenly the weight of everything I had been through, not only that week or that year, but everything that came before, as well as everything I would be going through going forward came crashing down. While I could not possibly know what was ahead, it seemed as if I could feel it. I also sensed God's presence even more deeply than I usually do. It was as though God was asking me a very serious question. I started sobbing again. I do not remember how long I cried, but I remember saying to God, "That is the one and only time I will ever feel sorry for myself, I promise."

Then I looked up and answered God's unspoken question, "Do whatever you will with me, but please let him live. And please prepare me for when you take him." And I *felt* God's answer and responded, "Thank You."

Everyone I know says that we are not supposed to "make deals" with God. In that moment, I knew we had a deal. A solid pact. "All" I had to do was love this gift and let God. I was different from that moment forward, so profoundly different.

I did not have the words to articulate how different I was then, but now I say only somewhat light-heartedly that I channel the Holy Spirit. I feel God's constant grace and presence in my life. I think that this is available to all who ask, and I am so glad that I asked. I am so glad I said, "Yes."

Are you ready?

Later reflection on this shows me that I have been looking for signs of preparation since Ryan was born. I have at times thought about what I will say at his funeral. What I will do when he is not with us. Someone dear to me pointed out recently that this is not a normal thing for a mother to think about. No, I do not suppose it is.

April 19, 1990

My Little Sweetheart,

It's been a roller coaster since your birthday with the ups reaching the clouds of Heaven and the downs licking the flames of Hell.

We found out Monday that you have extra "material" on chromosome 8. Although we don't know what exactly that means, it almost positively means problems for you later. I am so sorry.

I look at you when I feed you, and it is hard to believe that anything is or will ever be "wrong" with you. You are so sweet, innocent, and cuddly.

April 27, 1990

My dear son,

Today we found out that your daddy is a "balanced carrier" for your chromosome disorder. It's complicated, but basically your extra material on chromosome 8 is a result of material that broke off his 12 and trans located to his 8. Since you don't have any missing from 12, the condition is not balanced in you.

It was hard for us to hear last Monday; today we actually felt we got some good news: there is only a 10% chance of its happening again; you probably won't be autistic; and we can hold onto any positive signs since you probably won't regress.

You weighed 7 pounds at Dr. Marsha's visit and grew an inch and 1/4! These are positive signs, too.

We love you very much and are still hopeful that you will lead a full, happy life even if it's not "normal" – whatever that means.

All my love, Mommy

Maps of a different sort

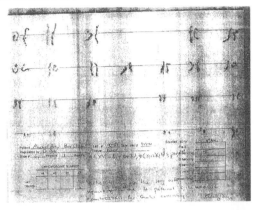

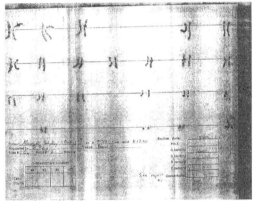

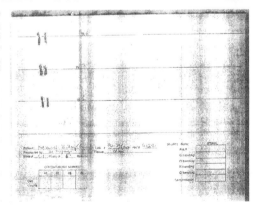

Eraser?

All these many years later, I still remember how I felt when I looked at these chromosome maps for the first time. The kind and patient Dr. Aslan was explaining the "extra material" on chromosome 8 that came from chromosome 12. It even looks small on the map, which, of course, is a zillion times bigger than it is in the cells — EVERY cell in Ryan's body. How can something so small cause so much damage? I had the strongest urge to get an eraser and erase the dark material that looked so much like a pencil smudge — **could someone PLEASE give me an eraser?**

I had that feeling because I wanted Ryan to be "normal" for *his* sake. For my own sake, especially after walking this journey as his mom, I would not have *ever* changed one thing about him.

November 25, 1990

My dear little "Pip Squeak,"

After reading Dorothy Butler's "Cushla and Her Books", I am inspired to pick up this diary again. I will try to recall the highlights of your seven-month life the best I can.

You are such a good baby. I can take you anywhere, and have. We have had you out with us to dinner many times, shopping – I even took you to a movie once and you only made a peep when you were hungry. So I nursed you and all was well.

I began calling you Pip Squeak affectionately very early. You were so tiny – until now. But, I'm afraid it has stuck. Everyone calls you that now.

Where do I start? I could kick myself for neglecting this journal, but there never seemed to be time or energy. So much has happened in your short life, there was only time to handle it, not much time to reflect on it.

Fortunately, much is recorded on your 'sticker calendar' and in pictures. The calendar is nice because it has a sticker for major events that we placed on the days they occurred. Perhaps I should sit down with it and use it as an outline. I will do that, but it is at home so I will stop for now.

Living Chaos

Shortly after Ryan was born, it was clear that my two "half" brothers, Steven and Brian, needed a home. Our mother had died close to Brian's 10th birthday, and while I wanted to take them back with me at that time, their father would not allow it. In 1990, when they were 16 and 14, they were desperate for some love and care. Larry felt strongly that we should take them in. While I appreciated the sentiment, I wondered if this was a desperate attempt to keep me in the marriage, as I had filed for divorce already. At first, I refused to consider taking them in. After talking to my brothers, I caved. They needed me. My divorce could wait. Their arrival shortly after Ryan's birth started a roller coaster that would end in a good deal of growth for me. I am grateful. I think my brothers grew some, too.

The stories about raising two teenagers in a bad marriage while having a special needs child could fill a whole book, but I will just say here that they both loved Ryan so much. There were times when I knew that without both of them I would not have survived. In spite of the craziness that was our weird family life at the time, we taught each other many lessons. We had battles and drama regarding drugs, alcohol, and girls. But we also had many joyous memories of them interacting with Ryan.

I am so grateful for them and happy that they are still part of our lives. Kiran still has a special bond with Steven, and both girls are close to Brian's family. Steven calls me monthly, knowing that I will always welcome him with open arms. I am more of a grandma (known as GranTi = GReatAuNtTerI) to Brian's children than an aunt. I am happy about that.

Desperation

This book is not about Steven and Brian, but the years they were with us coincided with Ryan's first three years, so they are part of his story. We had ups and downs, as do all families. It was always hard for us to decide whether I was sister or mom. As it was, the role of mom worked better in the end, but it took us a while to get there. I was not a perfect mother/sister to them, but I did love them perfectly. Loving is what I do best.

Early on, while we were still trying to figure out our roles, I saw an advertisement in the church bulletin for a workshop called "How to raise teenagers and live to tell about it." I thought it was just what we needed, so Larry and I went to the first night to register.

We arrived late and were told that the class was already full, but that another one was starting in four months. A panic welled up inside me, "We will not make it four months. Could we just stand at the back and hear the talks? We won't bother anyone; we'll just take notes." I must have looked as though I were going to faint because she said, "You go right in, we'll make room."

November 29, 1990

Dear Ryan,

Your first days at home were hard. You had to be in a clear "box" under the blue "bili" lights for jaundice. We could only keep you out long enough to feed, change, and take your temperature. A nurse came every morning to take a blood sample from your heel. Once, she took off the band aid and the blood stain was the shape of a heart. She said, "Ryan, you are so sweet, you even bleed in heart shapes."

Those days were difficult. But, I was so thankful that you were at home, it didn't matter.

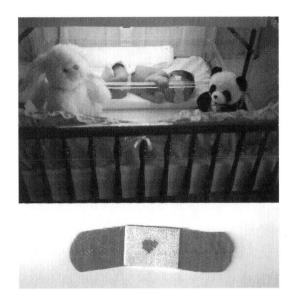

More Heart-Shaped Blood Stains

Circa April, 2013

This happened as I was packing the manuscript to send to a publisher that someone I cherish recommended. Truth is stranger than fiction.

Please, no one freak out about this. As Zulfi was unpacking the luggage he picked up today (he got in six hours early yesterday, so his luggage did not follow), he noticed a glass frame he had packed broke. He told Kiran, "Give this to Mom, she'll know what to do." Yep. Except I missed a piece, and it cut my pinkie.

No biggie, wrap it up and continue packing up the manuscript. Well, the wrapping fell off, and blood dripped off on the outside of the envelope. I wiped it as quickly as I could, and the smear is the shape of a heart. I smiled. Apparently, Ryan and I both bleed in heart shapes.

No way am I getting a new envelope. It's a sign. It's Palm Sunday, we all wore red (for the blood of the Passion), and it feels like I'm sending off my first born.

The book will be rejected, everything I write seems to be rejected the first time. That's OK. It's a start. And God sent me a blessing in the sign of a heart-shaped blood stain.

God is Good. (Of course, God is Life and Life is Good)

Christmastime, 1992

Dear Ryan,

We are at Aunt Trisha's in Texas, and I'm taking a few moments to write. I've been carrying this around for a while, but I never seem to have time to write.

Woops, I fell asleep. See what I mean? ☺

In looking back over your calendar, I see "surgery" marked for May 9. That was a very rough time. You had pyloric stenosis, which is the swelling of the muscle between the stomach and intestines. You lost weight the week before while they tried to decide what was wrong. It was so sad to see you in the hospital. I slept in your room – I couldn't bear the thought of anything happening to you. The hour you were in surgery was the longest in my life. I think if anything ever happens to you, they'll have to bury me, too.

[My friend, Zulfi, was with me during your surgery because Daddy had to be out of town.]

Mommy

Advocate

The definition of "Advocate" is the speaking or writing in favor of someone. It is what parents do for their children.

Many years later, I reflected on this journal entry and realized that Ryan's surgery at three weeks of age was the first time I stood up as advocate for him in our tangled journey through "Western medicine." I told the assistant, as respectfully as I could muster, that he was not going to draw any more blood from him until he called Ryan's doctor. While I am not a medical doctor, it was clear that Ryan was dehydrated, and, given that he weighed less than seven pounds, every ounce of liquid was important. The assistant was surprised but honored my wishes and went to call the doctor. I realized then that it was up to me to make sure doctors, nurses, assistants, and therapists cared for Ryan *under* my guidance. While medical professionals often know more about chemicals and reactions, I know the most about *Ryan*. The best caregivers we have ever had, and the *only* ones we ever keep, are the ones who have treated us as partners in Ryan's care.

January 7, 1991

My dear son,

I have tried to make time to write, but it is hard. "I'm so behind, I'm first!"

My times with you are the happiest of my life. You are so precious. When I touch your soft skin, I feel a bond that no one can break. You are my son! "Bone of my bone, flesh of my flesh." Part of me, yet separate.

I think I know why people go crazy over babies. Not only are they adorable and soft, but they are little for such a short time – you have to get your 'baby moments' in quickly. If theirs are grown, people must grab other people's babies when they can. It must be why everyone stops to smile at a baby, why everyone becomes friendly and helpful if I have you with me.

I love you with all of my heart, my precious baby boy!

Mommy

May 17, 1991

Dearest Ryan,

Over four months since my last entry. You are over a year old; so cute and so much fun. You are the single most joyful thing in my life. Nothing I have ever done or could ever do will compare to the joy of having you.

I met our child birth instructor in Burger King the other day. Her baby has Down's. So very sad. We are having lunch together today. Maybe we can help each other.

You are still not crawling, but you are doing many other things and your VSD has almost healed. You are a gift and every day is a gift. I hope God never asks me to return this gift.

I love you, my son.

Your mommy

Summer 1991

Dear Sweet Ryan,

We are in the airplane on our way home from a week in Florida on vacation. As usual, you were very good. You are hardly ever any trouble.

You are growing so big. Someone took my baby and gave me a little boy instead. ☺

You are also growing more curious. You want to touch everything and taste everything. But you still don't cry if I take something from you, and you never cry to taste something. You just show signs that you want it. It's so cute to watch you stick out your tongue or open your mouth and move towards whatever I am eating or drinking.

You are also very fun. You laugh and smile all the time and you are getting more vocal.

When we get home, I will give you your fourth haircut.

There is nothing or no one who has brought me more joy than you. I am the luckiest mom in the world to have you for a son. I only hope that your life is at least as happy as mine has been with you in it.

I also hope you are going to be this gentle and good as a man.

Love,

Your mommy

June 4, 1991

My dearest Ryan,

The house is quiet – a rare and wonderful occurrence. You are asleep and every-one is gone. I have this peaceful feeling that I am the luckiest person in the world. I have so many blessings – I need to count them more often. Somewhere along the way I changed from a positive, bubbly person to one who is negative more than I'd like. God and I are working on that. You make it easier.

I love you with all that I am.

Your mommeeee

AllOne

AllOne is the way I spell alone. The reason is probably obvious, but in case not, it is because I am One with God (All) when I am alone. I love to be alone. Blaise Pascal, the famous French mathematician (OK, the philosophers claim him, too) said, "All of humanity's problems stem from man's inability to sit quietly in a room alone." While that is perhaps a slight oversimplification, it has a great deal of truth. Throughout these letters to Ryan, I have noticed how I held on to my AllOne time to regenerate. It is when I did not get AllOne time that things fell apart.

June 30, 1991

Dear Ryan,

Even though you are "behind" in development, I have great hope that you will be a happy and whole person.

Yesterday your daddy brought you to work to see me because I hadn't seen you all day. You seemed so happy to see me! It made my whole day.

You have never crawled or done many other things babies your age should have done; you are not walking yet, but you brighten the lives of all those around you. You do have the ability to learn and love it when we clap and say, "Yay, Ryan" so I know you will go further than the doctors thought. And even if you go no further, you have brought more happiness to the world than most people have in a lifetime.

I love you!

Mom

November 11, 1991

Dear sweet baby boy,

Just now as I watched you get into a crawling position, I cried. [At 18 months, you still do not crawl or walk.] It is hard to describe the feeling as I watched you. Maybe I rejoice more in everything you do because we are not sure you will ever do all the "normal" things. Perhaps we also rejoice more because we all work so hard with you to achieve the developmental milestones. Because we have more pain, we have more joy.

Thank you.

Your mommy

"He will probably never crawl."

Reading this years later, I have only to close my eyes and recall the many times I strapped Ryan to a skateboard to build up the strength of his arms and legs. I almost always had tears in my eyes — it seemed so cruel. I only did it because I trusted the PT/OT who suggested it. I started this after one physical therapist had encouraged us to give up; "He's probably never going to crawl." She did not say you would not walk, just that our attempts at crawling were not working. Another doctor told me how important crawling was in development, so we should not skip it. I think this was the beginning of my questioning and seeking second opinions and new health providers when the ones we had "gave up." I was not about to give up. I cannot say what drove me other than faith and a fierce and relentless love, as well as a desire to help Ryan achieve all he can be. Now that we have two "normal" daughters, I feel the same fierce and relentless love, except most things are easier for them.

October 31, 1992

Almost a year since I have written in here. I have written much in my other journal.

Just now you and I were 'dancing.' You love for me to hold you and dance to music. The moments like these are, by far, the happiest moments in my life. I love you so much, my son.

Thank you for all the joy you bring to my life; the pure innocence with which you approach everything, the way you get so excited when you see me, the way you say 'Mama,' the look on your face when you first heard the book make the chirping sound – one of Eric Carle's books, *The Very Quiet Cricket*, and countless other precious moments ....

January 19, 1993

Dear Ryan,

A new year, a new president whose policies I do not think will work, but I still have hope that this will be a better year.

You are growing so big. You are still very well-behaved and very sweet.

From the moment you started growing inside me, until I saw your cute face, until I held you, through all the pain and joy, my love for you has grown and continues to grow. Each day I am amazed at the swell of love that wells up inside me when I hold your hand or read you a story or hear you laugh or watch you crawl "in the miritary style" (after the baby elephant in Jungle Book) or, like tonight, when I watched you sleeping ...

At times I think I have more love for you than humans can possibly give or receive. I hope I always love you the right way – using "tough love" when necessary.

Thank you, God, for giving me the strength to deal with a handicapped child and emotionally bruised teenagers and husband. Thank you for always picking me up when I fall, make mistakes or lose control. Thank you for helping me see the joy in the pain, the rainbows after the rains. Please help me to continue to learn from my special little boy – who truly is a gift from God, my very own angel.

Learning to see the Rainbows after the Rain and not to blame the Rainbows for the Rain

I have always loved rainbows. Come to think of it, I love rain, too, but not as much as a sunny day, especially one with a rainbow in it. Throughout my life, I have encountered many people who "blame the rainbow for the rain." The song "Never Blame the Rainbows for the Rain" is track #1 on the album Keys of the Kingdom. It was written by Ray Thomas and Justin Hayward and is one of my favorites.

More on Rain

I think I have always loved rain. I remember calling rain "liquid sunshine." And for likely as long, I have struggled with reign, in particular, the "reign or Kingdom of God."

I remember being asked to participate in a two-year certificate program for Mission Leadership. I am quite certain I was not the first choice since I was not yet in a leadership position in the Catholic university where I worked at the time. In fact, I am quite sure I said, "No" when first asked. Saying no to God does not work for me.

A colleague who became a good friend through this experience, Janine, helped me a great deal. I remember during our posts online, while reflecting on "the reign of God," that she told me, "I just think, instead, of the RAIN of God falling on everyone and making everything and everyone grow. I think of Kingdom as *Kin*-dom — the rule of the kinship." So beautiful. From that point on, whenever I hear "the reign of God," instead of imagining an oppressive patriarchal kingdom, I think of us all dancing in the RAIN of God — the *kin-dom* of God.

I suppose it is not surprising that one of Kiran's favorite quotes is, "Life is not about waiting for the storm to pass, it's about learning to dance in the rain."

Even More Rain

Just this afternoon, during a mindful meditation session, the instructor shared the acronym RAIN, which stands for "84,000 lessons" that include R — recognize (and absorb), A — accept, I — investigate (non-analytically), N — non-identification, "let it be." Perhaps it is through those steps that rainbows are made.

Kingdom and Reign/Rain Keep Following Me

This whole struggle with kingdom and reign followed me on an ACTS (Adoration Community Theology Service) retreat. The song for our group was "Build Your Kingdom Here." Well, about two nanoseconds after I heard the song, I remembered my friend's words and quickly got over my dislike of all things patriarchal. The song "Build Your Kingdom Here" by Rend Collective Experiment is wonderful. When I sing it, I sing "rain" for "reign."

Wanna Be

As I am adding reflections, I realize how much I am adding about singing and dancing, songs, lyrics and poetry. While I think Ryan's sisters received their gifts of music through me, this talent remains unskilled in me. I am just a "wanna be." But no matter, poetry, singing and dancing have always been a part of my life, and most especially after Ryan was born. More later on how Ryan and dancing saved me.

What is in Aunt Jenny's Tummy?

One of the most special moments I recall from the year when Ryan was five is his answer to the question, "What is in Aunt Jenny's tummy?" Aunt Jenny, which is what Ryan calls my dear friend, Jennifer, was finally pregnant after more than a decade of trying. We were all very excited for her and her husband, Uncle Bob.

Through the years, whenever Ryan and I saw someone we knew who was pregnant, I would ask, "What's in _____'s tummy?" Ryan would always say, "Baby." Ryan loves babies, and the look on his face when he said "baby" was so sweet.

I took Aunt Jenny to lunch once a week to cheer her, because she was housebound after her pregnancy became difficult. During one of those wonderful lunches, she shared with me that if the baby was a girl, she would be named Lindsey, and if the baby was a boy, he would be Benjamin. I never shared the conversation about names with Ryan.

The next time Ryan saw Aunt Jenny, he hugged her tummy. When we asked him the usual question, "What's in Aunt Jenny's tummy?" Instead of "baby," he surprised us with, "Ben." I almost fell over. He had not heard the name conversation, but somehow he *knew*, not just that Aunt Jenny's baby was a boy, but that he would be Ben. A few months later, Ryan greeted the baby boy whose name became simply "Ben," rather than Benjamin, which his parents preferred. *Ryan knew.* I truly believe Ryan knows many things that I have yet to learn.

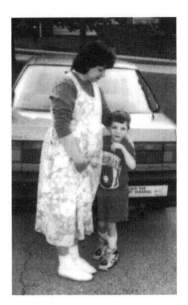

3

Stories of Life

All stories are true.
Some of them even actually happened."*
*A variation on James A. Owen's
"All stories are true. But some of them never happened."

Instead of a resume, a person in academia has a *curriculum vitae,* a story of life. I suppose in a very real sense, these letters and stories form a *curriculum vitae* — the story of our life with Ryan, which happily is ongoing.

Letters that came later

What's Wrong?

October 31, 1993

My good friend, Ruth, my three-year-old Ryan, and I had decided to brave the long line at Ryan's favorite fast food place because they were giving away free kids' meals.

Ruth and I were deep in a pleasant conversation with Ryan standing patiently between us, when I felt a tap on my right shoulder. Now, for some reason, being tapped on the shoulder *really* annoys me. I guess I would just prefer a voice to get my attention. I turned to see an anxious-looking woman pointing at Ryan, "What's wrong with your son?"

I looked down at the top of his head covered with thick, wavy chestnut-colored hair. He looked up at me just then with his big, round, hazel-colored eyes, encircled with long, curly eyelashes. He gave me that winsome smile that he reserves just for his mommy, and my heart sang. I turned back to the waiting woman and answered truthfully, "Nothing."

I turned to resume my interrupted conversation with Ruth, and it was not long before I felt the annoying tap on my shoulder once again. She seemed frustrated, "No, I mean what's *wrong* with him? What does he *have*?" Trying to hide my disbelief at her rude persistence, I looked again at Ryan, one hand trustfully placed in mine, the other holding a little yellow school bus, one of his favorite things. "He has a little yellow bus," I offered.

Turning around once more and resolving never to come to fast-food promotion nights again, I thought surely that would be the last unwelcomed remark from her. Wrong. *Tap, tap, tap.* This time I did not try to hide my annoyance. The woman did not notice or chose to ignore the look of exasperation on my face; she was annoyed with *me*. "I mean, *what does he have*? Because my niece has cerebral palsy, and she looks and acts kind of like him, so … and I wondered if that is what he has."

I managed to choke out, "No, he does not have cerebral palsy," just as, gratefully, the line had just moved so that I could turn from her and go get Ryan's "free" kids meal for Halloween.

The Most Interesting Things Happen in Line
May 18, 2013

My dear Ryan,

Today, nearly twenty years since I wrote that story, you and I had quite a different experience while waiting in line. You, Lauren and I went to our favorite "big box" department store. You were riding in a "wheeling chair," which is the name Kiran gave wheelchairs when she was three.

I was hanging out with you while we waited for Lauren to try on the clothes she wanted. A lady walked up to me, and I thought at first she was an employee since she had on the right color shirt. Then I noticed she was with her daughter who had just finished trying on clothes. This rather large, sweet woman with beautiful dark brown skin and eyes put her face close to mine and touched both of my arms. For some reason, this neither startled me nor bothered me in the least. She smiled at me, and I smiled back.

She started whispering, "At least you know where your son is. You know he's safe. You know he's not on drugs. He's not in a gang...." I looked at her sad eyes and responded without thinking, "And I know he's not fighting in Iraq or Afghanistan." With tears in her eyes, she hugged me, I hugged back. "How did you know?"

her eyes saying what her words could not. She continued, "People think folks like your son aren't in their right minds, but he has the sweetest mind and the kindest soul." We hugged again, and she walked away saying, "God bless you both." I'm not sure if she heard my answer, "God bless you, too, and I'll pray for your son."

Another Halloween that went very wrong
October 1997
My dear little one,

This story was hard to write as it was such a tragic and unnecessary event. This was an awful, life-changing day for all of us.

We were at a pumpkin patch. It was a cool, sunny October day and you and Kiran were having fun doing one of your favorite things, a hayride. You have always loved to ride – anything really, but the more interesting, the better.

It was time for your father to pick you up, and you didn't want to go. We didn't want you to go, either, but I talked myself out of the feeling of dread I had watching you go off telling myself I was just sad that you were going. I had to share you with your father after all. Buddy told me later that he had the same feeling of dread, and we made a promise after that NEVER to talk ourselves out of premonitions.

We got the call about 9 pm. "Ryan fell. He's at the hospital emergency room." I don't think I heard anything after that. I took the full flight of stairs in two steps, calling to ask Lisa and Eric to come get Kiran and for Zulfi to meet me in the car. On the way, I got a few details. Your father took you to an outdoor adult party. You fell from a second-story deck to concrete.

I ran from the car to the ER and was escorted to a small room, where your father and some lady were praying. "Please sit down and pray with us." I will not repeat what I wanted to say, but was too shy and nice in those days to actually say. "Where's Ryan?" Your dad responded, "They won't let us in there." I just left. With a calm that could only have come from God, I went to the front desk and said to the woman, "I am Ryan Maxwell's mother, and I want to see him, if you don't have the authority to let me do that, please go get someone who can." The lady opened her mouth to say something, looked at me and thought better of it. "I'll be right back." She brought a man who took me into the room where you were – as I walked in, the room started spinning. You were covered in blood and unconscious. I thought you were dead. I swayed. Larry appeared from somewhere, and I thought I might kill him, except it took all my strength to stay standing.

As soon as I touched you, you responded. The doctors looked around. Perhaps they would rethink the not letting mothers in the room policy. I tried to ignore Larry, but I am sure I responded quite angrily at a couple things he said because one of the assistants commented to another, "Divorced." I wanted to punch him. All this violent anger that I have NEVER felt before.

With the help of God, I ignored them all and just held your hand. If the doctors needed your hand, I moved and touched your foot. I never let go; I would never let go until God told me it was time. We had a deal. It was NOT time. I looked up and reminded God. Just in case. The greatest sense of peace came over me. No, it is not time, but it is going to be rough for a while. OK.

Fast forward to intensive care. We spent a week there. They would not let me sleep in your room, so I slept as close as I could and took vigil in the chair by your bed whenever I was not in the way. I learned so much about Medicine that week, and I learned that it was very important to be nice to the nurses because they are so critical in minute-to-minute care. I try to be nice to everyone, but it's easy to be crabby under this kind of stress.

You nearly died once because they gave you too much morphine. Once again, I came to your side, and you relaxed. We are connected. There were many bumpy moments, and not all of them had to do with medical care.

I loved your grandmother, your father's mother. She was a gracious lady and very kind. We got along very well. She of course adored you. She came to intensive care and after learning that you were "out of the woods" took on the grand-motherly job of chastising "us" for not watching you. I had never said a cross word to this wonderful lady, until then, I had never had a reason. I looked her sternly in the eye and said, "You need to give that speech to your son. Ryan was with him at a party when he fell from a second-story deck to concrete." I turned and went back to be near you. Somehow I think she continued the speech even though I could no longer hear it.

Buddy took your sister Kiran home to sleep. Sleep was far away from me, but despair and anger were close. So somewhere in the dead of that night, which is to say in the wee hours of the morning, I called Father Mike May. This was the first of many times he came or answered a late-night call.

He was first my professor in graduate school, then my friend. He is a Jesuit, whom he calls the sheep dogs of The Church, as opposed to the shepherds, which I suppose are the diocesan or other orders of priests.

He was later to become a very close friend of mine, and our whole family loves him. I call him Mikey, a name we gave him in graduate school as a play on the Life cereal commercial. Instead of "Mikey hates everything," as in the commercial, we said, "Mikey knows everything." (He is VERY smart.) Everyone else calls him Fodder May (another early Kiran-ism). He was the priest at Buddy's and my wedding, as you know. We have asked him to celebrate all of the sacraments for you and your sisters since your first communion. Our Parish priests have always welcomed him to participate. As a result, we affectionately refer to him as "BYOP" for "bring your own priest."

That night, that awful night, he held my hand for a very long time. He brought a rosary, but we just talked and prayed other prayers. He anointed you with the oil for the sick. It was not the last time.

As I have learned to do my whole life, when life gives me lemons, I make lemonade. So, we made the best of the situation, which was much easier to do after we knew you were going to live.

Two of the happy memories I have of camping out in intensive care that week are of nursing your baby sister Kiran and working out an important math problem.

Kiran was such a good sport and thought this was just a new place to play. She was happy to see you when we first brought her and glad to know where Mommy had been. And on the third day, when we knew you would be OK, I had Buddy bring my books – I was in grad school for a Ph.D. in math. I worked out one of the hardest problems I had been working on that later became the foundation for my dissertation. I give the credit to God for helping me tap into what I had just started to learn – meditation, being present in the moment, and changing focus when necessary.

You made it out of intensive care. But that was the beginning of sleepless nights and another issue that we were not yet prepared to handle.

Blame

As I look back these many years later, I can and do tell myself *theoretically* that anything can happen to children when we just look away for a moment. I can and do tell myself that there is no use in blame. I can and do tell myself that "there but for the Grace of God go I." I do try to focus on the good, such as the fact that once Larry dove head-first down the carpeted stairs to break Ryan's fall when he was just learning to walk, rather than wondering why he let Ryan be in a position to fall down the stairs in the first place. I am human, however, and I have not yet completely come to peace with the fact that he took Ryan from having fun at a pumpkin patch to an adult party where he fell down stairs again. This time, they were not carpeted; they were concrete. And Ryan's life — our lives — have been forever changed.

We spent the next several months trying to take care of Ryan and juggle life with a rambunctious toddler. Zulfi had a stressful job. Larry had a stressful job. I was in graduate school, no stress there. We were not always at our best, and I was angry with Larry much of the time because I did not think he was helping enough. Buddy said to me, "Let it go. Do you really want Ryan with him if he is too busy or too stressed to handle him?" It was like cold water on my face and warm water on my feet all at the same time, "Of course not, and thank you for reminding me of that." I had the most overwhelming sense of gratitude for Zulfi being willing to help me take care of Ryan when Larry was not able to.

We have come a long way since then, but we had not yet learned how to make the most of everyone's gifts so that Ryan would be the best he could be. I am happy now that Larry sees him often and is very happy to do so, and that we try to say, "Yes," whenever it works in both of our lives. It took us a while to get to this place.

The First Seizure

When I thought I could not take any more, my brother, Kenny, and his wife offered to watch Ryan and Kiran so that Zulfi and I could take a break. We went camping in Pere Marquette, a park in Illinois about an hour's drive from St. Louis. The park is named for Father (Pere) Marquette.

We were supposed to stay three days. During the middle of the second day, we had another premonition. Without even saying a word, we started home. As we drove, Kenny called. "I'm really sorry to bother you, but I think Ryan just stopped breathing for a minute, and his eyes rolled back in his head. We are taking him to the hospital." Kenny was witnessing Ryan's first seizure. "We're on our way. We'll meet you there.

At The End of Everything

As in the beginning of the well-known Patrick Overton poem, "When we walk to the edge of all the light we have," I was there. I have been there so many times in my life and in our journey with Ryan. I suppose everyone has. This time was one of the first and most frustrating navigations through Western medicine. At the core, the problems were a lack of communication and a belief that doctors should not be "bothered" with certain things. Ryan almost died.

Ryan had been sick with the "virus of the month." It was taking a harder toll on him, though. He had suffered through several seizures that night and morning, which meant no sleep for any of us. I made an appointment with our beloved neurologist, Dr. Garret Burris.

It was a fortunate thing, at least I thought, that this neurologist and our pediatrician were in the same building at the hospital. I took Ryan to the neurologist's office in Ryan's big comfy wagon that we had bought for his birthday. He loved riding around the neighborhood in it.

Dr. Burris checked everything, changed Ryan's seizure medications (again), ordered a blood test, and suggested that we see the pediatrician for the virus.

While in Dr. Burris's office, Ryan threw up. As I changed Ryan's clothes to make him more comfortable, I also tried to soothe an unhappy one-year-old Kiran. I was trying to contain the overwhelming fear and self-pity that threatened to swamp my emotions. Zulfi and Larry were both out of town. We had no family in town. I thought for the hundredth time that we should move to Texas near Gigi, Papa, and Janet.

I forced back the tears, rounded up Kiran, and pulled Ryan in his wagon to the pediatrician's office downstairs. I was certain they would fit us in since we needed to see Dr. Marsha. Plus, we were already there. I explained to the receptionist what was going on and asked to see Dr. Marsha. "She does not have any appointments today." I knew that if they got a message to her, she would see Ryan. I knew it. "Please just tell her we're here." I do not recall the receptionist's name, but she is no longer there. I am pretty sure I know why.

I decided to go downstairs for the blood test while waiting for them to get a message to Dr. Marsha. On the way downstairs, Ryan threw up again and started convulsing. I had already used his change of clothes. I felt myself coming close to "losing it." Instead, I called Jenny. She heard the pain and desperation in my voice. "I will be right there, and I will stop on the way and buy Ryan a change of clothes." She is, and always has been, an angel. While we were waiting, Ryan started convulsing again. I went back up to the pediatrician's office and asked if Dr. Marsha had responded. "No."

I do not recall who suggested that we admit Ryan into the hospital, because at that point I wanted to scream. It was probably my idea, because he looked near death. No one should see their nearly seven-year-old near death. I picked him up and carried him to the ER. He was blue. Jenny followed with Kiran, who was now in the wagon. Jenny's face showed the concern that was in every part of me. What followed was a blur of machines and a bustle of doctors, nurses, and assistants. I doubt that I had ever felt worse in my life than when I had to help hold Ryan down while they put an IV into his arm after he finally stopped convulsing. The look on his face ... "Please God, don't let that be the last thing Ryan sees."

It turns out that Ryan had a severe reaction to a medication that does not react well with one of his seizure meds. Because we were early in the process, the reaction was unknown to the pediatrician, and we got the medications from different places, so the pharmacy could not catch it. I now do my own research on any medication.

I later had a talk with Dr. Marsha about what happened that day. She had never gotten the message that we were there. She agreed that it was not handled well and confirmed my belief that she would have seen us had she gotten the message. She went part-time not long after that. I have always wondered whether incidents such as these had an effect on her decision or if it simply was a matter of wanting to spend more time with her own children. I would later come to a similar choice, much later than perhaps I should have.

That hospital is still my favorite hospital. Everyone was simply lovely. They took care of Ryan *and* me. They put up with Kiran and even asked Jenny if she wanted coffee. I have replaced the truly awful memories with these memories.

The Bad Guy

Perhaps most parents can relate to the feeling of being "the bad guy," the one who consistently applies the tough love and is the disciplinarian. I used to resent this role, until I realized I had some say in it, which is to say, it was, at least to some extent, up to me. I did not have to be the bad guy always. I started sharing the role with Zulfi and Larry as well as other caregivers.

As I reflected on the recent episode at the hospital, especially the part where I was needed to help hold Ryan down, I decided that I would not ever do that again if there were anyone else to do it.

I cannot recall many times when I have felt worse than when he was struggling with all his might to get away from people he thought were trying to hurt him, and I was "helping" them hold him down. The pleading look in his eyes was often followed by closed eyes and the deep "sleep" induced by anesthesia. I would slink out of the room and pray that that was not Ryan's last memory of me. This episode made me resolve, "Never again."

Shortly after making that decision, I took Ryan to a regular pediatrician visit, and the doctor shared that she was no longer giving the shots. Her reasoning made so much sense. "I need the children to feel safe with me. If all I ever do is give them a shot when they come, it is not good for trust." Of course, that meant the nurses and assistants had to give the shots, but there were more of them than there were doctors, so they could rotate.

It was interesting that this change in their practice coincided with my decision never to hold Ryan down while someone caused pain or discomfort to him, even though I knew it was a necessary, short-term discomfort for his own good.

Many years later, when we found the lovely dentist, Michael Hoffmann, he sweetly said to me, "Mom, we're going to give Ryan sedation now. I have four assistants if I need them. Why don't you go read your book, and we'll call you soon." Same philosophy. Wise one he is, Dr. Hoffmann.

It is OK for Mom to be the bad guy when Ryan needs to eat some broccoli, but when he falls asleep, I want the last face he sees to be mine, and I want us both to be smiling.

"The Woody Story"
Circa 2004

Ryan has never shown any interest in toys. He loves people and books, preferably together; he loves people to read to him. The Christmas after the first *Toy Story* came out, his younger sister, Kiran, got a Woody doll. Ryan took it. A fight ensued. This was new to us, because Ryan has never cared about anything. He gives EVERYTHING to Kiran. We bought Ryan a different Woody doll, but it was bigger than Kiran's, and he wanted nothing to do with it. We were never able to find one exactly like that one, although we and many of our friends and family members have tried. We have an odd assortment of some 12 or 13 Woody things. Ryan likes them all, but it is clear that they are not the "real Woody."

They had fought over "the real Woody" for almost a year before we were able to convince Kiran that the noble thing to do would be to give it to her brother. She reluctantly said he could play with it (as he had been for the past year), but that it was still most definitely *hers* because Santa brought it to *her*. OK, then.

From then on, it was Ryan's Woody but-not-really-it's-Kiran's (if she was within earshot). She finally decided she could part with the Woody doll she had hardly touched by declaring it "his" over the summer.

For a while, Ryan took it everywhere. It has all the characteristics of a well-loved toy, including busting seams and lots of dirt. His wonderful long-time teacher, Dennis, realized how much Ryan loved Woody and used him as a motivator for him.

During the school year, Woody spent most of his time at school or in Ryan's backpack. I thought I remembered Dennis sending Woody home at the beginning of the summer, but a couple of months ago, we could not find Woody ANYWHERE. I searched the attic playroom, all the toys in Ryan's room, and the girls' room. I tried to keep this low-key whenever Ryan asked for Woody, "He's got to be here somewhere ...."

I sent a note to Ryan's new teacher asking her to verify that Dennis sent Woody home. She asked him. He thought so. No Woody anywhere.

One morning, I went to get something out of Ryan's closet. I saw the soft luggage bag we used for Ryan's things when we traveled to my brother Brian's wedding in July. I specifically remembered bringing Woody and putting him in the accessible side-pocket so Ryan could get him whenever he wanted. I wondered if he was left in there. HE WAS.

Ryan was so happy! He actually danced with Woody when I handed the doll to him. He insisted on taking Woody on the bus, refusing to put him down. His teacher sent home a note that Ryan was so excited about having Woody back and had the best day at school that he has had all year. He even ate all his lunch!

When he got home, he wanted to call Larry and tell him that Woody was found. Now, Ryan is not the most articulate at speech, and when he says "Woody," it sounds more like Woory.

Larry could not understand what had Ryan so excited. I could see the very animated and oft times frustrated conversation from our side. "Woorry. Found Wooory." No, no, no, WWWWOOOOOORRRRR-RYYY. Found Woory." This went on for several minutes until Ryan took the cordless phone, put Woody up to it, and yelled, "LOOK!"

Channeling the Holy Spirit
Subtitle: How to Buy a Mattress

As many have heard me say before, "I don't just pray, I channel the Holy Spirit." I certainly mean no disrespect by this statement, and I believe that everyone who would like to can (and should) do this. What I mean by "this" is that I walk in constant, "please guide me" mode. If you ask, the Holy Spirit seems quite happy to guide you. The problem is that I do not always listen to the guidance. Alas, God gave us free will so we could be truly happy (which means we can also be sad). When I do listen to the guidance, Life is so good. Sometimes the goodness spills over, as it did in this instance.

Ryan had not been sleeping. Zulfi and I had resigned ourselves to taking turns sleeping on the trundle bed next to Ryan because nothing else worked. The problem was that the mattress was 16 years old and had no support. After helping Ryan into bed and then sleeping on the bad mattress, I pulled out my back and could barely walk. Because I wasn't working, and the State stopped Ryan's funding, we would not be able to afford a new mattress for a couple months. I called Larry and asked if he could help. Of course, he said yes. He even gave me the names of some places with good mattress deals.

As I was running two errands I needed to do before going mattress shopping, I passed not one, but three mattress stores.

I decided to visit the place where we had purchased mattresses for our girls over the past year or so. I did this not just out of loyalty because one of the places I passed was the same company; I did it because I was answering some strong pull. I rarely question these tugs any more.

Instead of the usual male sales clerks, there was a lone saleswoman. As I pulled into the parking lot, I could see, through the building's windows, that she was dancing. I smiled. She stopped when she saw the van, so I did not say anything as I went in except, "Hello." Then I explained that I wanted to check prices on a plain twin mattress. She showed me all of the options in my price range without any pressure. What a lovely experience. It turned out that we could afford one, and they could deliver it that day!

As we sat down to do the paperwork, she shared that she was a bit embarrassed about what she called 'praise dancing.' "Oh, you do not need to be embarrassed by that with me! I love to dance and sing, especially to upbeat Christian music." She was so relieved. I shared with her our retreat song, "Build Your Kingdom Here," and she wrote down the name and said she would look it up.

She went on to say that things had been so slow lately, and she felt she'd been unfairly "written up" for low sales. She told me that she had just said a prayer to the Holy Spirit to "send her some people." Not only do we always get an answer; but sometimes WE ARE the answer. I had goose bumps. What a lovely experience.

More Rainbows

February 21, 2014

Dear Ryan,

Today was one of those really draining days, a rainy day, but one with a rainbow.

Your yearly dental cleaning was scheduled for 8:30 a.m., arrival time 8, with meds to be given with water, instead of the usual applesauce, no later than 6:20 a.m. Katelyn, one of the morning caregivers, came and helped me get it all done, complete with an extra set of clothes and coaxing you to wear a short-sleeved shirt even though it was cold. The morning was a bit rough, but mostly because your younger sister, Lauren, was having a "teenager morning." After about the fourth warning, I told her "no sleepover this weekend." Things got a bit better after that (for a while) because she thought if she were nice to me, I would change my mind.

I dropped Lauren at school, and we headed to the dentist. Dr. Michael Hoffmann does dental work under anesthesia in his office. He is kind, compassionate and very good at what he does. The same is true of his entire staff. We were blessed to find him. The second year he cleaned your teeth I was lamenting out loud that we were going to have to put you under anesthesia twice that year because of the severe wax build up in your ears and your intolerance of having anyone touch your face and head, much less clean out your ears. He offered cheerfully, "I can do that for him while he is under." Really?! He has done it ever since. He is an example of what is right with Western medicine.

I do not suppose it will ever get any easier for me to watch four people hold you down so they can give you the gas that will help you relax so they can give you anesthesia. All that just to clean your teeth. Your life is so hard. You deal with so much. I feel so small complaining about how hard it is on me when you are the one who goes through so much.

Still, it was a hard day. Throughout the day, your sister was lobbying to get me to change my mind about the sleepover. I kept getting text messages on my phone with crying monkeys, other sad pictures, tugging pleas in hopes of negotiating a different consequence ... ugh. It took just about all of my strength to get through the day and NOT to give in.

Friday was your regularly scheduled day with Chris from AADD (Association on Aging with Developmental Disabilities). He decided it would be easier to keep the schedule and just help me at the dentist, rather than to find another time. And he was a lot of help.

There were bright moments in the day. I love holding you even though it saddens me that you have to be in such pain and go through so much. You were so cuddly and loving. As much as you love to be around Buddy, when the chips are down, you still prefer your Mommy.

I had made an appointment with the lawyer to discuss appealing the State's decision to drop funding of Sarah Care. Let me just say, it was a struggle to leave you feeling so tired and sore, even with your beloved Chris, to navigate the traffic and parking downtown, and to discuss everything with the lawyer. Even though the meeting was about as positive as possible, I was drained as I was heading home in rush hour traffic.

More texts from Lauren. Ugh. She was not giving up easily. I looked up to ask for some of God's strength. It took all I had not to stop at Cravings and treat myself to a meal AllOne (my spelling of alone, especially when I am being self-full, my term for what many call selfish.) I came home, checked on you, and convinced Lauren that she was not having a sleepover. After a good, long cry, she gave up. I asked her why she thought I had taken away her sleepover, "I need to learn to talk more respectfully to you, and I need to take care of the dogs without arguing." Good.

When Buddy came home, we all cuddled on the couch that pulls out into a queen-sized bed. I invited Lauren to lie next to me, and she did. We watched a feel-good movie, and I remember thinking as I lay between you and Lauren, that this was truly the best feeling a mom can have. Some days are just hard, like rainy days, and on those days, God seems to send us rainbows in many forms.

Sometimes the Hardest Thing is a Haircut

Dear Ryan,

You were born with a head of thick, wavy, dark hair. I love to run my fingers through it when you let me. You had your first haircut at 4 months and have had them about every month since then, except for a tough, rather long, period when you would not let anyone get near your face or head. I have memories of three of us holding you down while you hit and kicked just so we could get the hair out of your eyes.

Those years were tough, and not just because you would not let anyone cut your hair. It is interesting to me that I have put most of the pain of watching you go through so much out of my mind, and the one thing I remember is a special haircut. Then again, it was not really the haircut that was the most special.

We had taken you to the auxiliary unit of St. Louis Children's Hospital. I do not remember the name of the unit nor do I know if it is even still there. At the time, it was next to the hospital and served children who had needs somewhere between the emergency room and the full hospital. We needed to call for an appointment, but it could be the same day. You were usually out later the same day.

This time, the stay involved anesthesia. As you lay there deeply sleeping off the anesthesia, I thought, "Now would be a great time to give you a haircut." As I looked around the place filled with white beds and sterile equipment, I realized there was probably no way they would let me. I asked one of the nurses anyway. I seem to recall his name was Mike. He was a very kind nurse, and listened with compassion as I explained how hard it was to give you a haircut. I even told him the story of the last attempt. He smiled with compassion, but said, "I am sorry, but I cannot give you permission to do that." I am sure my sigh was audible.

A few minutes later, he walked back in, smiled at you sleeping, and put a towel and a pair of scissors about a foot away from me. Before he left, he added, "No one else will be here for an hour. Let me know if you need anything else." I quietly cut your beautiful hair, and took a luxurious moment to run my fingers through it. You even smiled in your anesthesia-induced sleep.

Mike must have been watching from somewhere because just as I finished and started to clean up, he came in and said, "I will do that." And he did. I could not thank him because that would acknowledge permission, but I hoped my smile said it all. I thanked God for nurses like Mike who really seem to understand how sometimes the hardest thing in caring for a child is a haircut.

Love,

Mom

Pudge Controls the Weather?

In the adorable movie *Lilo and Stitch*, a very distressed Lilo panics when she cannot provide Pudge (the fish) his daily peanut butter sandwich. When asked why this is bothering her so much, she responds incredulously, "Pudge controls the weather!" I love this movie, especially the music, and that is one of my favorite scenes. However, it has long been my belief that no one, not even God, and certainly not Pudge, controls the weather.

Some time ago, during the certificate program at Aquinas Institute, we were given a "gifts inventory" to take. This was done in order to ascertain what gifts the Holy Spirit has bestowed. Knowing I have been blessed and having felt for a long time that I "channel the Holy Spirit," I welcomed the test.

I was somewhat surprised, however, when one of my strongest gifts was "intercessory prayer." I began to pay closer attention to my prayer and the outcomes.

The morning of Ryan's 16th birthday party, though, I was not even thinking about it. We had invited over 100 people, and the party was to be mostly outside. We had scheduled carriage rides from 3:00 p.m. to 7:00 p.m. because he loves to ride in anything, really, but especially carriages. The forecast called for a 100 percent chance of rain all day.

I am not sure if what I said to God even counts as a prayer, and I did not even think about how it might sound to God. I probably even had my hands on my hips as I looked up, "I know You don't control the weather, but I know You *can*. I'm not asking for myself, and Ryan never asks for anything. He has a hard life, and he loves carriage rides. PLEASE."

It stopped raining at 2:30 that afternoon and did not start again until 7:30 p.m. My prayer of gratitude for my "weather miracle" after that was very intentional.

May, 2011

Dear Ryan,

Since I was a faculty member at a university with a speech clinic at the time, you were able to get services at the clinic for free. The director of the clinic asked me to speak at the dedication of the new clinic. Of course I was happy to do that. Here is a copy of the speech.

Dedication Speech Representing Parents and Clinic Clients

It gives me great pleasure to speak as a parent of a child who receives services from the university's speech clinic. I am especially happy that this talented group of people now has a brand new, state-of-the-art clinic in which to do their magic. If you have been to the old clinic, you know what this group has been doing and under what conditions. If you have not been, just imagine any of those stories you have heard or read of doctors trying to practice Western medicine in Third World countries with inadequate resources. They are simply amazing.

Anyone who knows me really well has heard me say that there was Divine Inspiration in my path to this university. One of the many, many benefits of working here at is that my son, Ryan, who has multiple handicaps, gets speech therapy at no charge.

He just finished his fourth semester, and from the first semester, everyone noticed improvement. He has not only added many words to his vocabulary, he is saying all of his words more clearly.

Well, there is nothing remarkable about that, you may be thinking, that is what speech clinics do. Ryan has moderate mental retardation and is 14 years old, well past the age when other therapists expected he would be able to add any new words or make significant strides in articulation.

In addition to the expertise of and superb care from everyone involved, Ryan and I have developed life-long relationships with those associated with this outstanding clinic. The director has given so much of her time to make sure Ryan's therapy works – from scheduling to end results. Each therapist and supervisor *becomes personally involved and attached, which is why I am sure that it all works so well. Quietly in the background, the director is there ensuring and enabling everyone to do what she does best.*

To give one small example of the dedication of this group, Ryan was particularly attached to a student named Katrina.

She always made him laugh and could get him to do essentially anything. She and Leah worked very well that semester to allow Ryan to grow a great deal.

Ryan has had bilateral casts on his legs since March to help him stretch his hamstrings. Whenever she had time, Katrina would follow me to my car with my three kids and help me put Ryan into the van.

I stand here before you a grateful parent. I am grateful to the university that allows my son to benefit from these outstanding therapists. I am grateful for the community that surrounds my son and me. I am grateful for the continuing commitment of this university to fund and support one of its most outstanding programs.

And now, Ryan has something to say. (I helped Ryan out of his wheelchair, he struggled to the podium. He said, "Thangoo." He received a standing ovation – and there were not many with dry eyes.)

Different Approaches

Growing up with two beautiful sisters has been quite the adventure for Ryan. As with every aspect of our journey with him, there have been fun times, tough times, and good lessons. There are many, many stories to tell about Ryan and his sisters, but I wanted to share something significant about the beginning of his relationship with each of them.

Our plan to introduce Ryan gently to Kiran, the new baby, did not work. Timing is everything. Unfortunately, Ryan was ushered into my hospital room while I was nursing Kiran. He looked at me as though

I had betrayed him. He was quite unhappy about this turn of events. However, he quickly came to love Kiran, and we have many pictures of Ryan holding and kissing her with his face beaming.

It was also interesting how Kiran responded to Ryan. From the beginning, she seemed to understand he was different and special. I will never forget when Kiran was about two, Ryan pulled her hair while she was trying to explain something to me. Without missing a beat, Kiran lifted his hand and moved out of his way, and continued her story.

About three years later, it was like *déjà vu*, except Ryan was pulling little Lauren's hair. He even hit her. Lauren's reaction was quite different. She looked at Ryan and sternly said, "STOP IT!" Then she hit Ryan back. Ryan has never tried to pull her hair or hit her again. By the Grace of God, I am thankful I had the wisdom not to "correct" Lauren for hitting him back and for seeming not to understand that he is different. She did understand but decided at the young age of two that pulling her hair and hitting her were still not OK. I realized then that he was to have two very different, but equally special, relationships with his sisters.

Big and Little

We have been watching shows about Barney the purple dinosaur for most of Ryan's life. Most parents endure kid shows because they teach good lessons, and Barney certainly does that. Thankfully, most kid shows have enough adult humor to make them bearable. Barney has none, in my opinion. If I believed in purgatory, and most days I do not, I think we would get a free pass from purgatory because of 20-plus years of watching or hearing Barney in the background. I say this in jest, well mostly.

When Kiran was four and Ryan was ten, they used to watch Barney together. She would sing all the songs and explain things to Ryan just in case he could not understand them. I can still hear her singing him the song about big and little that talks about being big and little, short and tall. It sends a lovely message that people come in all sizes. Some might say that Kiran got her notion of big and little from this, but I do not think so.

When she was five, someone asked her if she had any brothers or sisters. I smiled at her response. "Yes, I have a big brother. Well, he's not really my big brother. Well, he is, but ... well, he *is* bigger than me, but ... Well, he is my *big little* brother." She still calls him her big little brother to this day.

The Order of Things

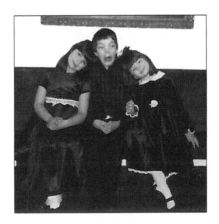

Dear Ryan,

It seems as though we are often talking about the order of things. Buddy has said to your sisters since they could talk, "The order of things is to finish high school, finish college, then get a job, then date, then get married." He sometimes jokingly changes the order and says that they should get married first, and then date. I wonder if he really is joking. So do they.

Mathematicians often deal with order. Most people think that mathematicians handle numbers much more than we really do. Most mathematicians deal with concepts rather than numbers, and when we are dealing with numbers, it is usually their theory, including ordinality and cardinality, rather than the numbers themselves. We do number our pages, which are essentially the only numbers in my doctoral dissertation.

As I was looking back through pictures to see which ones I should include in your book, I noticed something very interesting about the "order of things."

When your sister Kiran was born, Aunt Jenny gave me a very pretty necklace with two figures of kids made of gold with crystal birthstones for their bodies. The boy figure has a clear crystal for your birthstone representing April's diamond. The girl figure has a light green crystal for Kiran's birthstone representing August's peridot. I absolutely love it and wear it almost every day. In fact, I hardly ever even take it off. When Lauren was born, Aunt Jenny found a red crystal girl figure to represent July's ruby. Without even thinking about it, I added Lauren's figure to the right of yours so that the order was Kiran, Ryan, Lauren – peridot, diamond, ruby.

One day someone asked me why my kids were not in chronological order on my kid necklace. I had not thought about it, and answered, "I think it looks better this way." I do think it looks better that way, but I had not really thought about why, so I took a moment to do so. Perhaps the order I had subconsciously in my mind was girl, boy, girl or perhaps I just thought the colors looked better green, white, red. Kiran was about ten at the time, so I asked her what she thought. Without taking much time to think either, she answered, "Mom, that's the way we always are, around Ryan to help him." Kids are so smart.

And as I went through album after album, I realized she is right. Most pictures that have the three of you are in this order. I am so grateful for all three of you. I especially like this picture taken around Christmas time.

Love, Mom

Ready?

August 20, 2014

"To Be a Mother is to Forever Have Your Heart Walking Around Outside Your Body." I am not sure who first said that, but it is so true.

Ryan often asks before he does something, "Ready?" He understands the importance of preparation much better than I do.

There are no words. There almost never are adequate words for times of deep sadness or joy. Today is the day I realized that Kiran was actually going to leave — it should have been December when we heard she got early acceptance, but it took until March for me to realize acceptance meant she was moving to DC. Then I worked on getting myself ready. She is ready — I have worked very hard on that. Teaching her to think for herself, defend her beliefs, whatever they are. Celebrating the ones that are different from mine. Teaching her, learning from her. I am proud of who she is.

For months, we have been shopping, planning, working, getting ready. Today is her 18th birthday. She is a year younger than almost all of her classmates because the cut-off date for school was July 31. All of her teachers said she was ready for kindergarten since she could already read "chapter books" and was very social. I have often wondered if I should have kept her back — then I would have her for another year. But no, she was ready then, and she is ready now. I wish I were. I wonder if I ever would be.

I found myself in her almost empty room, sat down and lost it. Nearly drowning in a sea of tears, I heard Ryan calling. Kiran had been lying with him, trying to tell him that she was leaving. He does not understand, or maybe he does. I took Kiran's place, silently. For 24 years, I have held Ryan's hands. His soft, sweet hands. But as I lay on the trundle, I reached into the bunk to get his hand, and he put his hand over mine. Every time I tried to move, he held on more tightly. And after the tears slowed, I looked up into his smiling face. For the millionth time, I saw what I thought must be the sweet smile of God loving me. I am not sure why I got lucky enough to be Ryan's mom, but I am so grateful. I am happy to be Kiran's and Lauren's mom, too. I just wish they didn't have to go.

Tomorrow we will drive Kiran to DC and on Saturday leave her there. I will leave a part of my heart there, but tonight Ryan reminded me it won't be my whole heart.

Other Angels on the Earth Masqueradin' as Humans

Then there are the wonderful caregivers who have come into our lives. Ever since the time I stopped taking Ryan to an arrogant doctor who did not give us good care, I took courage in the realization that I was a better judge of doctors, therapists, and babysitters for my son than anyone else, and we have never had another instance like that. I am happy to report that the good caregivers are self-propagating. Get one good one, and she gives you another who gives you another ... Jeanne has been the root of most of the wonderful caregivers in Ryan's life now. I am so grateful.

These caregivers are like family and say the most meaningful things. In the same category of "see what love can do," (explained later) I recently heard a comment that I will never forget. That morning I was getting ready to do Plan A when I got a call from Sarah Care, the wonderful place where Ryan spends a good part of his week. Nurse and Director Kathy called to say, "Ryan seems off. He had a slight tumble, he's not hurt, but he's asking for you." So, even though I had not even showered, I went. I checked him out; he was fine. I gave him the choice to stay or come with me. "Mommy." OK, Plan B. Later, I called Nurse Kathy to let her know that Ryan was OK. She opined, "I guess he wanted to be with the person who loves him the most." Yep, that is me. Glad he knows it.

A Recent Reflection on Plan B

Just took our dogs out for the last time tonight. The snow has covered everything, once again. I heard the voice of God saying, "Every once in

a while you need to know that I can cover it all and make it white again, make you slow down, stay inside and cuddle, work on Plan B ...."
It is all Good. God Said.

Reality Check
Circa September 2014
Some days are just plain awful. And then you get a reality check.

After teaching a(nother) frustrating class (the lazy whiners seem to be poisoning the class), I got a call that Ryan is "green," clammy, and "out of it." Indeed, he was. Since he had a seizure last week, I wasted no time getting there.

Our wonderful homeopathic MD's office said they would squeeze us in so we didn't have to do urgent care. We did wait a long time, which was hard because I had pulled out my back helping Ryan, who was very unsteady. Then Ryan threw up while we were waiting for Dr. Eastling. He threw up all over himself and the "wheeling chair." Sigh. I was feeling pretty sad for Ryan and even a little sorry for myself.

I had just barely gotten Ryan cleaned up when Dr. Eastling came in, checked him as thoroughly as Ryan would allow, and then diagnosed a virus. Nasty little, evasive bugs, those viruses. At least we get to go home and don't have to go to the hospital.

As we were checking out, we could not help but overhear a woman who could not afford $24 for her medicine, which insurance did not cover. My pity party disappeared. At least I have meaningful work (even if many of the students are lazy and it is only part time) and at least I can afford Ryan's medicine when insurance does not cover it, which is often. Reality helped put things in perspective.

Ryan had already perked up, and I knew as soon as I was home with my heating pad, I would too. The woman stepped out to go to the restroom. Together Ryan and I gave the assistant the $24 to give to the woman for her medicine. "Please don't tell her." We left so happy to be going home and to be able to do a small thing to help this lady. It really seemed to perk Ryan up as much as it did me.

The woman must have guessed, because as Ryan and I were struggling to the car, she came running out and hugged me. Neither of us said anything. At least not in words.

Life is Truly Good, even when it is hard.

Smile Anyway

I have received a lot of support and encouragement to write this book. The first thing most people said when I left my full-time position as professor and chair was "Good, now you can finish your book about Ryan. That book needs to be written." A couple people asked if I intended to put in pictures. So many of them said, "People just have to see his smile. That smile is amazing." One smile in particular seemed to capture a lot of hearts. Taken by a special caregiver from AADD after he and Ryan went to the Cardinals game, this one is "a winner." It captures Ryan's spirit so well that it seemed only fitting to put it on the cover of this book. Thanks to Christopher Labanca for taking it and allowing me to share it.

Questions I Never Thought I Would Have to Ponder

I have been fascinated with genetics since first learning about it in my high school science class. The science of DNA was new at the time since it had not been that long since Watson and Crick made their discovery. I recall thinking "this makes so much sense," while most of my classmates struggled with chromosomes, genes, and eye-color maps. My mathematical research also led me to deepen my study of DNA. Having a son with a very rare chromosome disorder led me to study even more. Knowing why something is the way it is, however, and doing something about it are two very different things.

Recently, my husband, Zulfi, asked me to read an article on the Web entitled, "Discovery provides evidence that the genetic defect responsible for Down's Syndrome can be suppressed." He said someone asked him what he would do if he could "erase" the extra chromosome and make Ryan "normal." I reminded him that chromosomes are in EVERY SINGLE CELL in our bodies. He asked, but what if they could? The question caused me to flash back to the moment I first sat in Dr. Aslan's office. Still in pain from the delivery of this beautiful baby, I stared in disbelief at his chromosome map. How can something so small — just part of a chromosome — make such a big difference? I had the overwhelming urge to grab the paper and erase it. Then I recalled that we have these 23 pairs of chromosomes in EVERY SINGLE CELL in our bodies. Cells are very small indeed and contain the even smaller, but powerful, chromosomes each made up of thousands of genes.

Today, 23 years later, I do not even need to think about my answer. Knowing what I know now, I would never erase that part that makes Ryan so uniquely Ryan. I would not have changed him then, and I certainly would not change him now. For a moment, I tried to wrap my head around what changing a 23-year-old mentally and physically handicapped adult into a "normal" adult would mean. How would it happen even if it could be done? Would he emerge knowing that he did not know how to read instead of still enjoying being read to as an adult, for example? Would he understand that he is "too old" to watch *Mr. Roger's Neighborhood* instead of loving it? What would he look like? Would his "deformities" disappear? I could not even imagine it. I realized I would not do it even if it became possible in my lifetime, so I stopped wondering how the transformation might occur. Seldom have I felt such a strong sense of relief.

I also felt a strong sense of gratitude, mixed with a good deal of hope, that this is not something we will need to consider. I am fairly certain, however, that this is not the last hard question stem cell research will bring up.

Pandas.

Pandas, they are so cool. They embody diversity — black and white merged together in the cutest, most inviting being. Chubby and happy, yet very fierce. They are Zulfi's favorite animal. I think he told me this soon after meeting him. I bought him a cute stuffed panda not long after we became friends. He named him Charlie. I have no idea why. For a special birthday years later, he said I needed a panda and bought me a lovely gold panda coin made into a necklace. When Ryan was born, he brought him a baby panda, that happened to hold a pacifier. Of course, we named him "Baby Charlie."

When Ryan was being weaned off his "binky," he found Baby Charlie, and we have the following pictures ...

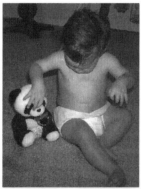

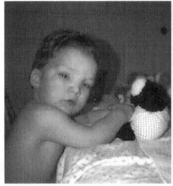
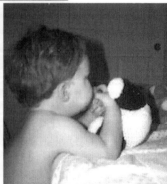

What's The Matter With You?

Circa 1998.

For a very brief period, it was necessary to have Ryan and Kiran at a day care center a few hours a day. It was not a pleasant experience for any of us, but there were some bright moments.

One of them occurred when we came to get Ryan one afternoon. We found him hovering around a group of young boys trying to be included. Ryan is very affectionate and loves to hug and kiss. His love is unconditional, and he expresses it whenever and wherever he feels like it. There was one boy, Robbie, who was very kind to Ryan, and as I came to pick Ryan up, I saw Ryan give Robbie a very warm hug and kiss. One of the more macho-type boys, Jake, laughed and tried to make fun of Robbie, who, without skipping a beat, said incredulously, "What's the matter with you? It's Ryan."

There had been so many times when I wanted to say to those who stare, to those who make fun, to those who ask the most probing questions, "What's the matter with you? It's Ryan."

Thanks, Robbie, for having the childlike faith and love, and the courage to express what we often struggle to express as adults.

Empathy and Sympathy

One of the most surprising things to me throughout my journey with Ryan is what people "feel sorry" for. Long ago, I stopped being so judgmental, I stopped getting angry, and few things people say even annoy me these days. It is even rare for me to get upset when someone "just does not get it."

Still, I think any book about Ryan's journey needs to include a reflection on sympathy, empathy, and feeling sorrow. Ryan's father recently reminded me of a discussion we had long ago about our problems not being worse, per se, just different.

One of the first and most unexpected instances of an expression of sympathy came when we were staying with one of my brothers, and I was giving Ryan his seizure meds. Since we were traveling, I had put all the bottles in the bag and had to divvy out some 13 pills. To make it easier for Ryan, we always fed them to him with applesauce. This had the added benefit that we snuck in some calories, because he rarely ate breakfast and is usually too thin. We have done this twice a day for years. For some reason, this evoked what seemed to be a deep sympathy for us from my dear brother. He reached out to me and said, "Your life is so hard, not sure how you do it." I thought, "If you only knew," but I smiled instead.

Another time was when we had someone we knew well babysit on what I thought was a rather uneventful night. She reported to her mother how "very difficult" our lives were and how challenging it must be to raise Ryan. From what I could tell, the most challenging part of the evening was that Ryan was still in diapers as a teen and had to be fed.

These are two people I know well and love. They mean well. They reached out to me in what they thought was something difficult in my life. These are two of many instances that make me realize that most of the time none of us really understands how difficult other's lives are; and even when we do, we really do not have the first clue of what triggers outbursts and pain.

Knowing this makes me try hard to give everyone the benefit of the doubt. If someone is crabby, I think, "Perhaps they had no sleep last night. Who knows why?" If I get cut off in traffic, I try to think something such as "Perhaps their spouse just said s/he wants a divorce." Insert your own scenarios and responses. Please do. Life will be easier. It does not matter why our lives are difficult; almost everyone's life is hard at least some of the time. Just love people. It will come back to you. Even if it does not, you will still feel better, and the person you are kind to will feel better, too.

Related to Empathy and Sympathy

I find it really discouraging when I hear someone say, "I sprained my toe," and the response is, "You think that's bad? I have a broken ankle."

Again, insert your own examples of this kind of exchange; I am sure there are many. There is no question that a broken ankle is worse than a sprained toe, at least for most people. Regardless of the scenario, someone in the world is likely to have it worse (or better). That does not mean we do not deserve to be heard and hugged when we sprain our toes.

Recently, a friend shared some frustrations about her work, and then checked herself and said, "I'm sorry you never get enough sleep … and … your life is so much harder." I told her that I hoped I would always be the kind of person and friend who can listen to others without comparing what they are going through with what I am dealing with.

For one thing, we are all different. We have different pain thresholds and tolerances. We have different experiences, different likes and dislikes. I am quite sure there are many people in the world for whom a sprained toe is as bad as a broken ankle. I am quite sure there are people who could go through certain challenges I have had with much more grace. I am hopeful that I have gone through many challenges with added grace as I have learned more. I do know that the friends I have, those who listen to my struggles and whose struggles I am happy to listen to as well, have made all the difference.

A Final Thought about Empathy and Sympathy

There have been many times when people have shared that they feel sorry for Ryan and for us for the hardships of dealing with a handicapped child. However, I have never felt that I needed pity, not only because of the joy that Ryan has brought, but also because of the many loving, caring people Ryan has brought into my life.

Among the many people I am privileged to know because of Ryan are our wonderful neighbors and fellow parishioners, Allen and Linda. "Mr. Allen" takes Ryan riding in his Porsche about once a month during good weather. We have often been the recipients of such loving care and generosity of time. After the first ride, we took a picture and wrote the caption, "No one is feeling sorry for Ryan right now." This was exactly what my girls said because they were very envious of their brother who got to ride in their dream car. "Ryan is so lucky," and they meant it.

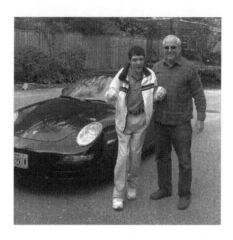

Suffering
October 2013

We grapple with many difficult questions as humans. I am often asked why God would create Ryan, a person who suffers so much, or why God would "make" Ryan suffer.

Long ago, I grappled with the question of suffering with the help of a good counselor, Beth, and a good friend, Rabbi Ruth. They both recommended the book written by another Jewish rabbi entitled "When Bad Things Happen to Good People." The other helpful book was written by my hero, and possibly favorite author ever, C.S. Lewis, entitled "Mere Christianity." I processed the books, all our conversations, all my experiences and came to a rather simple conclusion. God gives us free will in order that we can love God freely and can be truly happy. Puppets are neither free nor truly happy, after all.

In addition to the human condition of being biological beings in a finite world, as a result of everyone's being free to make choices and decisions, we get suffering. When I choose something you do not like, or when someone else chooses something truly evil that affects many, there can be suffering. The resulting chaos is complicated, but the reason for it is rather simple. We are free to choose Good or Evil. The collision of these choices often results in suffering. Sometimes there really is not much choice involved. Accidents and deviations of nature are part of God's creation. Sometimes the consequences cause suffering, and sometimes they cause joy, often both. I have learned that I have a lot of say in how I meet suffering. I am not sure where I heard it first, but pain is what happens to you, suffering is the story you make up about it. Recently, I had the following interesting reminder.

Last summer, I attended a monthly meditation group Sunday afternoons with my friend, Jeanne. I have learned that meditation is a great augmentation to my Catholic faith, and I am glad to be participating in this with these great women. One Sunday, the teacher asked us, "What is the gateway to compassion?" I wanted to answer, "suffering," but did not because I was not sure. When she answered her own question with, "Suffering is the gateway to compassion," I thought, "Of course it is." Why did I doubt myself? I know that. Christ helps us make good out of suffering, and compassion is one way Christ does that. At least that is my experience.

Life is Good, even when we suffer.

From One of Ryan's Morning Caregivers

In response to a Facebook post about Ryan's suffering and how it affects people: "What about the fact that no one can meet Ryan without being changed in some way for the better? I signed up to work with a young man whom I hoped I could help in some small way, and, instead, I feel like I got all the benefits. He "accidentally" spreads joy everywhere he goes … whether in the way he knows no stranger or even how he finds joy in the simplest of things: school buses, counting trash cans on the way to day camp, even stop signs. I think Ryan inspires everyone whom he meets and then seeks out joy in all of the small things that God has given us. His smile is like a spark that ignites that joy. He is truly a blessing, and I feel so grateful for all the time that I have gotten to spend with him." – Kari Miller Muskopf

The Girl Ryan and Other Wonderful Ladies

These lovely morning caregivers who are OT students self-propagate. Once, this resulted in MISS Ryan Jackson coming to our house. Kiran's sarcastic response made us all laugh, "A girl named Ryan taking care of our brother Ryan? Oh, that is not going to be confusing at all." Miss Ryan quickly endeared herself and was well worth any confusion that having "Ryan taking care of Ryan" caused. Somehow, whenever I said "Ryan," they each knew by my tone whether I meant my son or The Girl Ryan, which we used when talking about her to others. I am grateful that The Girl Ryan is still part of our lives. In fact, we are in touch with almost all of the people who have come to take care of Ryan in the mornings (Mallory, Kari, Justine, Katelyn, Elizabeth, Tess) by either the occasional pizza outing or other visits, phone calls, or Facebook.

Please and Thank You, November, 2013

Everyone compliments me (and Ryan) on his good manners. One of his first words was "than-goo" for thank you. While it would be easy for me to take credit for teaching him these and other polite terms, I did the same things with my girls, but they did not always stick. I believe that Ryan came to the earth understanding "please and thank you" and their proper responses much better than the rest of us.

Tonight while lying with him, I was reminded of how often I have said "thank you" to him. While holding his still, soft being, I reflected on his response, which has always been the same. Not surprisingly, it is not the same response that the rest of the world gives.

A while back, our beloved Jeanne lamented that the world responds "no problem" when we say, "thank you." She said this bothered her on many levels. To say "no problem" seems to indicate that a problem was anticipated; that somehow inherent in a person's helping another, there is a problem. I completely understood. I have not said "no problem" since.

Then I thought about other languages of which I know a little. In French the response to thank you (*merci beaucoup* = thank you A LOT) is *de rien* (of nothing = it was nothing). In Spanish, the response to thank you (*gracias* = in gratitude) is the same, *de nada* (of nothing = it was nothing). While I somewhat understand that the response to expressions of gratitude should be to say humbly that what I did in response was small, I ask, "Why do we do we reduce it to nothing?" The response to an abundance of gratitude (*merci beaucoup*) seems like it should be an enthusiastic, "I was so happy to do that for you because I love you — you are **so welcome** to my deed that represents my love." The short version of that seems to be "you are welcome," which is what we used to say when someone said, "thank you."

Even with many years of coaxing from me, lessons from Special School, and hours of speech therapy, Ryan struggles with articulating many words. Tonight, as with so many nights before, I held him close and said, "Thank you for letting me be your mom." He hugged me back and said the short version of the above, "Welcome." The fact that it was so clearly articulated made it all the more special. I think he understands that I know he fell straight from the heart of God, and I hope he knows how grateful I am. His "welcome" seemed to say that he knows it is so much more than nothing.

Disability Panel

For many years, I taught at a small Catholic university. I was asked one semester to be on the panel for parents of children with disabilities. This was part of the series of events during the semester dedicated to the theme of disabilities.

I opened my presentation by reading "Welcome to Holland" by Emily Perl Kingsley. This lovely article is something that seems to have followed me throughout my life, even long before I had Ryan in my life.

It is a beautiful reflection of a person whose plane landed in Holland instead of the planned trip to Italy. The point of the story is the importance of being happy where you are. If my journey with Ryan has taught me anything, it is the importance of being present and being happy where you are, even if you wanted to visit the exciting city of Rome, but instead are "stuck" looking at windmills and tulips.

I just want to say that I do not recall ever wanting to go to Holland, and I am still hopeful that I will one day get to go to Italy. I am happy to be wherever I am, even if I do not get to go to Italy, and still would be happy if I never go to Holland.

Neighbors are Accidents. Friends are on Purpose.
Sometimes the best of friends are the outcome of accidents that we purposely cultivate, like Eric and Lisa.

We had heard they were moving in, replacing the "pink flamingo" neighbors. However, we had not met them yet. Coincidentally, I met Lisa in a baby goods store a few miles from our homes. Our girls, just five days apart and nine months old, reached out to each other, as did Lisa and I. It was the beginning of a forever friendship. How ironic that next-door neighbors met in a store miles away. We were the kind of neighbors who had keys to each other's houses (not that we ever locked them, and they were free to walk in whenever) and, more importantly, to each other's hearts.

There are so many stories to tell, and I will likely tell at least some of them, but one of the first needs to be the bed.

A handicapped child has many "issues," as do all children I suppose. A graduate student has many, as well. The intersection of them is most assuredly a lack of sleep. Some of this is unavoidable, but we had reached a breaking point and decided that we needed to do something different to tackle the lack of sleep problem in the household. After two years, sleep center intervention and many drug trials later, I gave up. About this time, our dear friend and neighbor, Eric (Lisa's hubby), started making bunk beds.

I hate cages. I do not even like cribs. I had a hard time even putting our puppy in a crate, so you can imagine my reaction when the doctor suggested a huge crib for Ryan, who was about seven at the time. I was tired (pun intended) of not getting sleep and was worried that Ryan was not safe at night. I decided to ask Eric to build us a bed.

Eric patiently reviewed my sketches and said, "Yes, I can make Ryan a bed." He only charged us the bare minimum to build the "crib in the middle of a bunk bed" that would save us. The bed was a very sturdy two-bed bunk with a pullout trundle bed that would serve all three of our children for several years and serve Ryan for years after the girls outgrew sleeping with their brother. The middle bed where Ryan slept was a crib that could be locked for his safety and later just a bed with partial rails that he knew would keep him safe.

Years later, when we decided that we had to move closer to the city, Eric installed the bed in our new house. These wonderful people who accidentally became our neighbors most intentionally became the best of friends.

New Neighbors, The Murphys

We made the tough decision to leave our good friends and neighbors, Lisa and Eric because we spent most of our time driving. We became "house poor" to live in the wonderful neighborhood of Webster Groves, where one can walk or take a short drive to almost everything.

Since we were not used to home repair and this house was over 100 years old, it was like being cast in the movie, "The Money Pit." While Kenny was helping us move in, he pulled me aside and asked, "Did Zulfi lose his job?" Much of the house was blocked off; it was cold and dreary, and he could not see what I could see — the "potential."

Kiran resisted the move a great deal. She did not want to leave Jessica (Eric's and Lisa's daughter). To punctuate this point, she put a picture of Jessica and her dressed in tutus in the middle of what was her new bedroom, threw herself on the floor, and declared, "I am all moved in." No surprise that she was very involved in theatre in high school.

I was drawn by what I sensed would be a good neighborhood and a good place for all our kids to grow up. The previous owners are a lovely couple, the Harts, who had raised six kids there. Before we bought the house, Mrs. Hart had me over for tea to discuss the house and its rich history. We discovered that we were both math teachers, giving us an instant connection that has lasted many years.

I jogged their mail over to their new home for a year; it was not far away, and it seemed easier than dealing with the post office. When we discovered that it was finally time to worry about locking bathroom doors (no need for details here, I'm sure), Mrs. Hart brought the skeleton keys that were accidentally taken when they moved.

Shortly after we moved in, the neighbor across the street, now known as "Aunt Pam," brought over brownies. She said simply, "Welcome to the neighborhood. We are best friends with the former owners. I'm the kind of neighbor you can call at three in the morning, and I mean it." And she did mean it as we soon discovered.

Shortly after we got settled, Ryan had a bad seizure in the middle of the night. Zulfi was out of town. I asked Pam to come sleep on the couch in case Kiran or Lauren woke up, and she did not hesitate. What a gift Pam and her husband Peter have been.

It took us longer to get to know "Uncle Peter." He is quieter and sometimes seems kind of curmudgeonly. For some reason, Zulfi could never recall his name, calling him Jack Murphy. We would often have these "who's on first" kind of conversations. "What's his name? Murphy?"

No, Mahoney. "Jack?" No, Peter. "Oh." So he was "Peter Mahoney, also known as Jack Murphy" until we got to know him better.

Peter has a soft spot for Ryan. He always made time to stop and talk to him if we were out, and it became a tradition for Ryan to sit with Peter on Halloween. It was quite a picture: Peter sipping on Guinness and Ryan happy as a clam watching all the kids in their costumes.

This past Halloween, both Pam and Peter had to work late. They tried to opt out of Halloween. Pam had sent me an email to let me know, but I did not get it. Unfortunately, I had encouraged Ryan to eat by saying, "As soon as you eat, we will go see Uncle Peter." When I explained this to Pam, they dropped everything as soon as they got home and said, "Bring Ryan over." We found some candy and Peter made a big deal about putting it in Ryan's bag. Ryan was happy. I think Peter was even happier.

Neighbors on the Other Side

We shared our side yard with neighbors who had a son Ryan adored. He loved to watch Isaac, whom he called "Idack." Whenever Isaac was outside, Ryan would call "Idack, Idack, Idack" until we took him outside to watch Isaac swing on the tree swing (his yard), shoot baskets (our yard) or bounce on the trampoline (our yard). Isaac was very sweet and patient with Ryan, and never minded his being out there. In fact, I think he liked it even though they didn't talk to each other much.

Isaac is very intelligent, which was evident from an early age. He loved to tell stories involving science, science fiction, and history. We loved hearing them. One special day, we invited Isaac to lunch, and he said, "Yes!"

Sadly, after Isaac graduated from high school, his family decided to "downsize" and move. Isaac made a special point of coming over before they left to "hang out" with Ryan. Happily, we are still in touch. We recently met Isaac and his dad for ice cream.

Such are the neighbors we have had.

Sharing

When Jeanne invited me to be on the panel to discuss disabilities for the Occupational Therapy students at Washington University, my "yes" was instant. I would have said yes anyway to almost anyone, but the fact that Jeanne has been my dear friend for years, has saved Ryan's life, has provided me with so many good caregivers, and started the self-propagating pool of morning caregivers (from this same lot of students), made the "yes" instant and enthusiastic.

The panel was made up of a lovely woman who had cerebral palsy, an incredibly strong married couple who were living with the husband's lung cancer recovery and me in my role as Ryan's mom.

After we each had shared our stories and perspectives of "life with a disability," Jeanne invited the audience to ask questions. I was surprised that most of the questions were directed to me. I suppose I should not have been since many in the audience would be dealing with people like Ryan and their parents. One astute student asked directly, "What advice would you give us?" It was one of the many times when I called on my direct line to God, "Please answer for me, God, and don't let me screw this up."

Two things come to mind:

1. While caring for a person with disabilities, remember that he or she is part of a family. A wise doctor I know (Dr. Enrico Stazzone) once said, "If it doesn't work for the family, it won't work for Ryan." You will likely become part of the family, and it is important to keep that in mind.

2. The other is to speak to the person with the disability directly. So many times, caregivers have talked to me as though Ryan was not in the room, as though he is not a person. Just because he cannot express himself fully, does not mean he does not understand.

The panelist with cerebral palsy strongly echoed these thoughts from her experience. Once again, I was humbled to be a part of something that might make things better for those who are differently-abled.

Out of the Mouths of Babes in the Midst of Chaos

There have been so many times when Ryan and other children have made me laugh aloud and have relieved even intense stress. There have been many times when the perspective of Ryan or another child has made all the difference between "losing it" and "hanging on." While the following story is more about my great nephew than Ryan, it is an example of how Ryan has made me smile even during times of intense pain. And the look on Ryan's face upon hearing this was, as the cliché goes, priceless.

Mommies are Important

When you have 23 beloved family members in your home for days, there are bound to be many "moments." Some will be funny, some will be silly, some will be sentimental and, occasionally, a little drama will be thrown in to spice things up. I am so fortunate that my extended family gets along. They all help. Several can cook, and everyone is always there to say, "What can I do?" We are usually arguing about who is going to pay for this or that, which I think is much better than feeling taken for granted, and a sign that we are reaping the benefits of our hard work.

My family members really are so much fun to be around, and Ryan is always so happy when they visit or we visit them. I will admit that it is a bit of work having all the extra people in our house, but it is such a small thing compared to the joy that is present when they are here. As the year goes on, I am sure I will be writing reflections of our time together, but for now, there is one story that cannot wait.

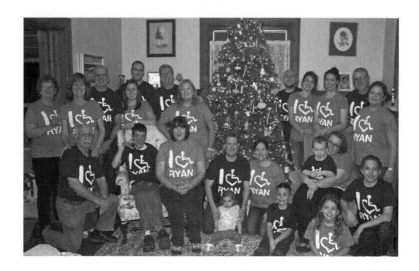

Most people who know me know that I almost never get to operate in "Plan A." I am not even sure why I make plans anymore; they rarely work out. I operate so often in Plan B that I think it is the norm. Almost as often, I am in Plan C or D and even Q or Z. During one visit, we thought we would drive through a local park to see the Christmas lights put up there every year. This was already Plan B since our first restaurant choice did not work out. When we arrived at the park, we discovered the line to get in was too long. Everyone was OK with waiting until the next night to try again, even the kids. Little two-and-a-half-year-old Liam took it in stride and decided to enjoy the Christmas lights he saw on the way home. Watching Liam get so excited about the lights helped Ryan perk up after having had two seizures earlier.

As we passed a beautiful lighted manger scene, Liam excitedly exclaimed "Baby Jesus!" We all took a moment to be grateful that this well-parented child reminded us of the reason for the season. The sweetest moment came when his mother, my niece Christina, asked him, "Who is holding baby Jesus?" He did not hesitate, "*Mommy* Jesus." Mary is smiling in Heaven right now, of that I have no doubt.

Helping and Serving

It is perhaps not surprising that Ryan has taught me so many lessons. It might be surprising that he has taught me the most about help, helping and helplessness. I know a lot of people who refuse to let others help them; I probably used to be one of them. We often view receiving help as a sign of weakness. Ryan happily and gratefully receives help from all of us. Some would say he has no choice but to receive help, but we all have a choice about doing it happily and gratefully. He seemed to know that instinctually.

One night, as I was helping him up the three snowy steps to the back door, his bright smile and "Thangoo, Mommy" warmed my heart. Later as I was making dinner, something he loves to "help" with, I asked him to get something out of the pantry. He seemed to be struggling, so one of his sisters offered to help. "No, ME!" He insisted on helping Mommy because he loved to and knew that he could. He eventually did get the item from the pantry, and then he struggled to carry it to me. I conveyed my genuine happiness that he was able to help in the form of a thank you and a hug. He was so pleased.

I have always known he is more intelligent than he can express and that he is very wise. Ryan has a very clear sense of when to accept and when to give help. As with most things, it is quite simple. You receive help when you need it. You give help when you can for someone else who needs it. It is usually better for both sides to be happy and grateful for it. I am happy and grateful that he helped me learn that lesson.

When God Asks, the Answer is "Yes"

I think this song captures the idea of humble helping service very well. Although I have never spoken about the "deal" God and I made, this song embodies the question God asked me so long ago and my "yes."

The Servant Song, by Richard Gillard, talks about knowing when to serve, but perhaps more importantly, the more difficult task of having the grace to let someone else be your servant, too.

"Giving Back"

I hate the expression "giving back," although I do not think I have ever told anyone that. Until a recent conversation with Zulfi, I was not even sure why. I have always been a giver, even when I have had very little to give; I would share. I do not say this with any conceit, it is how I am hard wired by the Grace of God, I submit in gratitude. I work hard and enjoy giving. As I have shared elsewhere, I grew up very poor, often doing without even the bare necessities. I have worked hard for everything I have. I would not have it any other way.

The first time I heard "give back," it was from a wealthy woman who had never worked outside the home. She felt that she owed something to society for that privilege. I decided just to be grateful that she was giving and did not think too much more about it.

Now the phrase is very popular as almost everyone says it. We are encouraged to "give back" to all kinds of charities. It pops up in all kinds of stories, in recruiting for volunteers and at schools and churches in all kinds of ways. Every time I hear it, I cringe. Deep inside a little voice says, "Give back? To whom? No one has ever given me anything. I have worked for it, and I give. Period. Not back." Of course, it is not true that no one has ever given me anything, but I certainly thought that I gave much more than I got and certainly more than my share.

Because we have worked hard, we have achieved slightly above a middle class lifestyle. We are between "middle class" and "rich," and this has meant that we pay much more than our share of taxes. Because of the U.S. tax structure, there are fewer options for families who actually earn a middle to upper class income. If the people who spend our money were better stewards of it, this would not bother me so much. I certainly am happy to contribute to roads, defense, and to those who truly need help, especially children in need. They do not seem to be the ones getting our money, though.

Instead, not only do I often not have enough money to pay for things Ryan needs, but also we are not eligible for certain services because we make "too much" money. Many of those services are not available otherwise. Some reward for working hard, and helping parents who can take care of one of society's truly vulnerable. As I usually do when something bothers me, I accept it as a lesson I need to learn and just sit with it, pray and listen.

There have been a few rare times when I have received so much that I do feel like I am "giving back." One of those times was during an ACTS parish retreat. This life-changing retreat has brought me 50-plus friends, who are more like sisters and has indirectly saved our marriage. So, when my name was called to serve on the next team, I said yes. I also agreed to give a talk. This is all very time-consuming. We have weekly meetings on Saturdays (before God wakes up), weekly meetings on Wednesday nights, plus the four days for the retreat in June. When Zulfi asked me why I said yes when I really did not have this much time to give, I did not even think about my answer and said, "I need to give back." His quick response was, "I hate that expression."

Not really surprised I answered, "So do I; I can't believe I used it. Why do you hate it?"

"Because it sounds like you stole something and need to give it back."

There is the lesson for me. While I did not steal anything, since everything on ACTS is freely given, I do have "it" and have grown from "it," and I need to give "it" back. With God's help, I hope to do that.

As part of the retreat team building, we each selected a wooden heart from a bowl. Each heart had a word from the gospel to serve as each person's theme for the retreat. When I turned over my heart, I saw that my word was "bestow." There it is again. Give. God, really, I do not have issues with giving. Are you asking me to give more? As a mathematician, I have learned how important definitions and assumptions are. I was assuming that the definition for bestow was give. I decided to look it up in the dictionary. Give is one of the synonyms for bestow, but it is not the first one. It is about the eighth one. One of the first definitions is "present." I submit as evidence that the Holy Spirit guides this process. I had just read the definition of bestow where the word "present" jumped out, about five minutes before the director called to ask me to present my story. There is only one answer to such a direct call.

Collegium

Collegium is an organization that has a summer colloquy for professors and administrators who are part of Catholic colleges and universities. The colloquy is entitled Faith and the Intellectual Life, and it does an excellent job of helping with the many challenges that are a part of academia, especially at faith-based institutions. It has the very best of both a seminar and a retreat.

I was asked to go to this colloquy during a time when I was struggling with being a professor and being Catholic at a Catholic university with mostly non-Catholics who seemed to be against all things Catholic. Later, I was asked to be a mentor and to share my experience. The talk is a reflection of the struggles I had at the time, especially juggling career and children, a struggle common to most parents today.

Collegium Mentor Talk

For this talk, two mentors are asked to tell the story of their calling as intellectuals and Christians. They explain how they see a connection between the spiritual and intellectual in their work and everyday lives and what fueled their sense of vocation early in their studies and careers. Finally, they discuss how they see their role as teachers of the church and/or teachers for the church.

Here is what I shared.

I recall several years ago when I sat where you are and heard Karen's (another mentor) story. I laughed until I cried; I cried until I laughed again. It was such a meaningful story that touched me so much that even when I heard it again two years later, it still had the same effect.

So, when Tom, the director, asked me to share my story on my "life and calling as an intellectual and a person of faith," I wanted to say, "No, I couldn't possibly do that; I'm not that funny." I had actually texted Tom in the airport "no," but the message came back. I guess I gave the wrong answer, so here I am. I promise I won't even try to be funny.

There are moments in all of our lives that have such a profound effect that all we have to do is shut our eyes and we can relive them, every detail and emotion flooding back as deeply as we first saw and felt them. We remember exactly where we were when they happened, what we were thinking and feeling, even what we were wearing. For some in the room, the assassination of President Kennedy was such a moment, for probably everyone, the crashing of the Twin Towers might have been another. And, of course, there are the happy ones: the birth or gotcha day of a child, the reconciliation of a loved one, finding something precious that was lost.

For me, one such moment was the first time I heard, "Ryan's mom is here." The little girl who said it was announcing my presence at a party at Ryan's godparents when I had to arrive late. Ryan, who was still a baby at the time, was already there. The little girl, who had not yet met me, made this announcement as though I were someone really special because I was Ryan's mom, and everyone needed to know that I was there.

This was profound for me, perhaps somewhat, because Ryan has a rare chromosome disorder called partial trisomy 12. It is so rare that it is not even listed in the National Order of Rare Diseases. In fact, he has the only recorded manifestation of this disorder in medical literature. As a result of it, he is moderately mentally and physically handicapped. Finding this out when he was born pushed me into the realization that the childhood development books would not help. I decided to throw out all the books and "just live it."

Hearing this little girl announce me this way reminded me that this was an opportunity to let God use Ryan to help the world. To my extreme gratitude, more people have seen how special Ryan is rather than seeing his handicaps. I have always been a spiritual person, but this was a turning point in my life like no other.

Having Ryan also made me realize that the usual 9 to 5, pressure-filled job was no longer an option. I had always loved teaching when I got to do it as part of my job in computer-related fields, so I went back to graduate school and got a Ph.D. in the field that was my first love, mathematics. (My bachelor degree is a double major in math and computer science.) My first thought was that I would be happier doing something I love and that teaching would allow me a career that had more flexibility. That has turned out to be mostly true. Getting there was another story.

My long journey to a Ph.D. in mathematics started after my divorce from Ryan's dad, Larry. While we share the parenting of Ryan, most of his care is with me. This alone would have been enough responsibility. However, the untimely death of my mother made it necessary for me to take in two of my younger brothers. Then, when Ryan was three, I sent him to a special school. Time marched on, and other milestones occurred, such as my marriage to Zulfi (called "Buddy" by Ryan) and the birth of our two daughters. Still, I studied. There were many ups and downs during that time regarding Ryan's health and growth. These were difficult years, but they are also among my happiest because I was doing everything I loved: caring for the people closest to my heart, studying math, and teaching. I felt very lucky indeed.

When I finally graduated, I realized there was no place for me in St. Louis. Washington University does not usually hire graduates from Saint Louis University. Saint Louis University does not usually hire its own graduates full time. The University of Missouri – St. Louis did not need anyone full time, nor did anyplace else it would seem. I felt pretty lost until Fontbonne, a small Catholic university, advertised for a position in computer science. I had left that world, but I needed a job and wanted to teach, so I decided to give it a try.

After three years of re-immersing myself in computer science and working on average 80-hour weeks, I was so burned out that I decided this was not what I signed up for. I had already typed my resignation letter when the current dean asked me to go to Collegium. It sounded luxurious to be away from my hectic life to reflect on faith and the intellectual life, so I said yes. I had no idea what was in store for me.

The entire week seemed choreographed and magically masterminded to heal me and keep me in academia. I remember spending long periods in the chapel praying about vocations and asking God to help me "belong." I took part in everything, from listening to the speakers to playing whiffle ball. I tried to listen. I met some amazing people with whom I still keep in touch. The most important thing that happened is that I was reminded over and over, and in multiple ways (I can be slow sometimes so God was not taking any chances here), that teaching is a rare opportunity to touch lives. Teaching at a faith-based university gives us freedom to do that in ways we would not have in any other vocation.

I came back, tore up my resignation letter, and asked the chair for a compromise. "Please let me teach one math class, and I'll continue to do this CS stuff." She agreed. Since then I have worked to achieve a better balance so that I can truly do what God called me to do, and that is to be open to letting him guide students through me.

Collegium may not be as profound for you as it was for me, but I encourage you to take part in as many activities as you can and to listen. Be open to what has been carefully choreographed for you this week. It may just change your life.

A New Gold Standard for Happiness

The following story is only tangentially related to Ryan. His story is not complete without stories of his sisters and their friends and stories of how I learned to be happy in a life with many challenges. Everyone who knows me well knows that I hate to drive. If I were rich in money, I would have a chauffeur. No one was happy when Lauren was told she had to leave the school she loved, the school she had been at since the age of three, the school THAT IS TWO BLOCKS FROM OUR HOUSE. She was mad at ME, as though it were my fault. I was not too happy myself.

Her new school is 30 minutes away. Fortunately, we found a carpool, which divided my driving by three. Our carpool consisted of two lovely boys, adopted from Guatemala, one very sweet, shy Irish girl (Addy) and my very angry Lauren. Most of the time, I just drove and tried to forget about life.

One day deep into the second year, Lauren and the boys were complaining about PSR (Parish School of Religion = CCD Confraternity of Catholic Doctrine = Catholic Sunday School for "Publics"). One teacher offered incentive for reading the Bible.

Somewhere in the middle of the conversation about PSR and the Bible, Addy, who rarely said anything, piped up. "The Bible. **Seriously**. I mean, are there any HAPPY stories in the Bible? *Seriously?* I mean, *Snoopy Skipping Happy stories. Seriously.*"

I nearly ran off the road laughing. For Christmas, my brother Brian surprised me with custom-made Snoopy skipping, happy tee shirts, and he even made one for Addy.

I told this story at Collegium and folks loved it. True stories from kids are the best.

I Believe; Please Help My Unbelief

As I am lying here on the trundle bed with Ryan for yet another night, many alternating with Zulfi for months of sleepless nights, it became clear to me that somewhere along the way, I started listening to everyone who thought they knew more about Ryan than I did. He stopped listening to music. He stopped sleeping. He did not like being touched.

Tonight as I lay next to him, I touched his hand, which he clasped readily, and he listened to me sing the whole Chaplet of the Divine Mercy, over and over … Eternal Father, I offer you … soul and divinity of your beloved son (I think Ryan resonated with that) … and those of the whole world. For the sake of your sorrowful passion, have mercy on us and on the whole world. Over and over … Ryan allowed me to touch him and sing to him. So, I did. Over and over.

I had the overwhelming sense that I needed to write this down and asked him if I could get my journal. "I'll wait," he said. This statement came out as clearly as when he said, "Welcome" to my comment, "Thanks for letting me be your mom." He doesn't say everything clearly, but when he does, I am listening. Ryan came to me for the sake of the whole world. I am grateful.

Diversity and Style

This is a story that, on the surface, has more to do with Kiran. Her views on diversity, as well as many other issues, have been affected by our journey with Ryan, and I think it is important to include them.

Since "Buddy" is dark, Ryan's two sisters are, too. So, they often get "counted" as [insert the current politically correct term for brown skinned people.] But in our family, we have every kind of diversity: religious, cultural, racial, as well as ability. So, periodically one of us will get annoyed at other people's seemingly limited views regarding diversity, namely that it is just about skin color.

Once, when we got a (well-intentioned) letter from the diversity committee at the girls' elementary school addressed "Dear family of color," a very indignant Kiran asked, "Mom, is white a color? You and Ryan are the only white people in our family. Are you invited?" Unsure, I called to ask. That was an interesting conversation. I went to the "diversity" meeting, and the school never again addressed the letters to families "of color."

Much later, a seventeen-year-old Kiran and I were chatting about diversity again, in particular, how different cultures dress. And that conversation led to a conversation about style, or, as Kiran would probably say, my lack of it. We were poor growing up, so I never got to dress in the latest fashions. By the time I could afford the latest styles, I opted for comfort rather than fashion. Actually, to be fair, I am nearly certain that I have never cared about wearing the latest trends. In fact, I recall not buying twisty beads in the eighties because everyone else was wearing them. I do like to think that I have developed my own sense of style and that I do dress OK.

As a transplanted Irish daughter of military parents who moved a lot (27 times before I was 13), I grew up all over, but mostly in the south, which seems to follow me everywhere. Many of the funniest clashes between the girls and me involve my "Southernisms." I can usually reduce them to tears just by singing hymns from my Protestant years. Of course, while singing, I revert to my "native tongue" — Southern.

During this funny conversation, I got the deep revelation regarding my notions of style, but Kiran just walked away laughing.

" ... They were buying them like they're goin' outta style," I said.

Kiran paused, "You know, Mom, you say that often, and I have NEVER understood it."

Me, "What?"

Kiran, "The phrase 'buying them like they're going outta style.'"

Me, "Oh, it just means folks are going to buy a lot of them."

"Yeah, but if they're going out of style, why would anyone want ONE, much less A LOT of them?" wondered Kiran.

Without hesitation, (I suppose I should be embarrassed about this), I explained, "Oh but that assumes you care about style. If it's about to go OUT of style and you like it, you need to buy them all up, so you have enough until they come back into style."

She just rolled her eyes and walked off laughing and mumbling, "Of course, I knew that."

It's Not Like It's Hard …

From the moment she was born, Lauren has been our "different drummer." And from the moment she punched Ryan back after he hit her, she has treated him just as she treats anyone else. This has developed into a sweet bond between them.

I love her view of Ryan, which is, "everyone has stuff to deal with …" and of the whole world. I also love her unique style of dressing, especially because she loves sparkle. Once, when she was about seven or eight, we were driving in the snow, and the sun came out causing almost everything to sparkle. She piped up from the back, "It would seem that God agrees that the world needs more sparkle."

On another van ride, much later when she had begun to have trouble with school, I was worried that we would not have time for her to finish her homework given all the errands we needed to run. She reassured me, "It's OK, Mom, I've done all the hard stuff, I only have math left." My child, after all.

Both girls have been a huge help with their brother, which often includes babysitting. This usually involves at least one diaper change and the giving of medication. Sadly, it can also occasionally involve the handling of a seizure. So, when we asked 14-year-old Lauren if she would watch Ryan so we could go out to dinner for Valentine's Day, she said, "Yes." When I asked if she was sure, she calmly replied, "Yeah, Mom, of course, it's not like it's hard to watch Ryan."

It's Not Like It's Hard … A Later Reflection

Some of the wonderful women who have read the draft of this book and offered constructive criticism have commented that I did not really share enough about how difficult it is to have a handicapped child. I have thought about this, and I echo Lauren's sentiment, "It's not like it's hard." Yes, it's hard to go through much of what we have been through, namely: ER visits, holding Ryan down for shots, his fall, his struggle for every milestone, changing diapers for over 24 years, wondering if he is happy, his frequent seizures, all the literal blood, sweat and tears, and the almost constant lack of sleep. It's all there. Focusing on those things is not who I am though. Yes, I do sometimes complain and share with good friends. I hope they do not mind too much.

I am frequently reminded of the joy Ryan brings into our lives. It's usually the little things that make me smile. Thank God yet again that I have Ryan to show me how easy gratitude can be. It's in those special moments with him that any pain I might be feeling from some unpleasant experience washes from my being, leaving behind a shiny, happy heart with more love inside it than I ever thought possible. The following story is a great example of this.

One night Ryan awoke at 3:00 a.m., scared, wet, and discombobulated. I was on the trundle next to him and held his hand. That was the last of my sleep for the night, but I was so happy to be next to Ryan.

As I put him to bed the next night, he said as clearly as he could, "Sleep well." I knew that was Ryan's way of saying, "I love you, Mommy, sorry for last night." How can I focus on the pain of the night before when I hear that?

I am so happy that I have written more about the rainbows than the rain. But rain is necessary for growth; I do not want to negate it. God's grace has helped me to look past the effort and see the joy; I am so grateful. The rain is so important, but the rainbows are beautiful. Do not blame rainbows for the rain, and do not forget to enjoy their beauty.

On the Bright Side

I always try to look on the bright side. Most of the time I succeed. As I hope the reader has noticed. and for reasons explained above, I have written mostly positive stories. But, of course, there are negative ones. I usually suppress those, or I do the only thing I can do, I look for the lessons for me. Thank you, once again, counselor Beth.

It would be a lie if the reader were left with the idea that this journey was a merry skip down some yellow brick road. There are times when, no matter how wonderful the caregiver is, I have wished we did not need a non-family member in our house early in the morning to get Ryan ready — or late in the evenings for physical therapy. It is an invasion of privacy even though I know we would not survive without the help.

Boundaries get crossed. Conflicts happen. After many years of having various "caregivers" and "health care providers" in our home, I have concluded, "People either come to love us and feel like family or they leave right away." It might be a slight oversimplification, but not by much. I am grateful that 99 percent have come to love us and feel like family. I'm probably equally grateful for those who have gone away, but, as I said, I try to look at the bright side.

Susan Hofmann, Ryan's PT (physical therapist), has come every Tuesday and Thursday evening for over a decade now. While I would love to tell you that it has been conflict-free, I would be lying. What I need to share is that she has become a sister to me, and there is no one else I trust more with Ryan's care. However, as much as sisters love each other, sometimes sisters have issues. She loves Ryan like a son, treats us all like family, and is one of the strongest living testaments to Christ that I have ever known. I love her unconditionally, and thank God for her every day. Ryan would not be walking or even alive if not for her and Jeanne, who gave us Susan.

In addition to the many years of care she has given us, Susan spent over 10 hours in the operating room when Ryan had his 15 orthopedic surgeries, because they would not let me be there. I am grateful that the wise Dr. Enrico Stazzone advocated for Susan to be there for us. She said her reason for doing this was to be able to care for Ryan better, but I am sure at least part of the reason was because she loved us. All of us. And she answers a higher calling.

In addition to evening physical therapy, having the morning caregivers come get Ryan ready has been a lifesaver. It has helped us sleep a little later, has helped our backs, and has made life better. It has not been without conflict, either. The first time I realized what having a person come into our house before 7:00 a.m. might mean was when we were interviewing the "next crew." Four young men answered the email ad. Um, that's not going to work with two teenage daughters who wander to the bathroom in all manner of dress (and undress). I had to send the email, "I hate to sound gender-biased, but we need young ladies."

Then there are the diapers. We always seem to need diapers. I was a recycler before it was popular. Being poor growing up, my family saved, reused, and recycled, and no one had to tell us to do so. We needed to. We used cloth diapers because the other kind were too expensive. That was cloth diapers without the service. We rinsed them in the toilet and washed, dried, and folded them. So, I didn't give it too much thought when my babies were born. I used cloth diapers because it was not only what I was used to, but it was also cheaper, it seemed better for the baby, and the environment. Had I given it any thought, I still would have done so because it is the right thing to do. Even during the worst of times, *e.g.* dysentery that followed our trip to Kenya visiting Zulfi's family, I still used them.

But Ryan is 25 years old and still "incontinent." I can't even tell you when we switched to disposable diapers, but he was in school. I apologize to no one. We had had enough, quite literally.

As odd as it may sound, while the State does not give us money for much else, we do get diapers once a month. Bryan is in charge of that. He makes sure we have diapers when we need them even when I give him very little notice. He embodies everything good in customer service. He does it with a smile every single time. He is on "speed dial" on my phone and has never once made me feel bad for texting or calling when, once again, we are out of diapers because someone forgot to tell me we were low. Bryan is a real gem, and while providing us with diapers for a decade may not seem like much of a claim to fame, it is the small things that make all the difference. He feels like a brother to me. He has shared part of his life story with me — such are the joys of crossing boundaries.

The main point of this story is that, when inviting or accepting (because you have no choice) caregivers into your home and life, you have some choices. You can set strict boundaries. There are advantages and disadvantages to that. If you relax the boundaries, there can, no there *will*, be issues. Relaxing the boundaries brings sisters and brothers. Sisters and brothers bring joy *and* pain. In my opinion, having a sister and brother with the occasional conflict is much better than having strict boundaries. How others handle these relationships is their choice. This is what works for my family and me, at least most of the time.

The Zulfi Story

When raising a child with disabilities, there are people who, inevitably, make comments that are annoying, puzzling or both. At the top of my list are the comments what many people have said about my husband, Zulfi. "It's really amazing that he loves Ryan so much." I look at them incredulously, but say nothing. What I am thinking is, "Really? Do you know Ryan? I do not know anyone who *does not* love Ryan, and I do not *even want* to know anyone who could not love Ryan. I certainly could not love or be married to someone who had trouble loving Ryan." I think that, but say nothing.

I think they really mean "it is hard for a man to love another man's child." Again, I think, but do not say, "Really? I love all children. Sure, there is a special place in my heart for my biological children, but I am pretty sure I would feel as much love if they were adopted." Does that make me different? I do not think so, but so many people say it, that perhaps it does. I find that sad. Ryan is the easiest person in the world to love, almost always. I want to scream sometimes, "It's not like it's hard to love Ryan!"

Perhaps if these people knew the whole story, they would understand. When I met Zulfi, I was married to Larry. While our marriage was challenging most times, I deeply believed in the vows I'd stated at our wedding. I wasn't necessarily happy, but it was my life then. The best part about our marriage was, and is, Ryan. I am grateful that was the outcome of our union.

I had met Zulfi before Ryan was born. I will never forget the day. I was working at Washington University Medical School in the biomedical computing facility concentrating on a genetics database project. My back was to the door, but I felt this intense energy when he walked into my office. I was afraid to turn around. When I did, I knew why. People talk about love at first sight, so this must have been love even *before* first sight. I have never had such an intense feeling. I remember thinking, "He is a work of art." Then he started talking in this lovely "colonial British accent," and I was gone. I am quite sure I did not hear a word he said; it sounded like music. He would later tease me, "My dear, I speak English the way it is meant to be spoken; you have the accent."

The intensity of my feelings scared me. As a result, I was not very nice to him. I told him that I did not handle the databases, which was a lie, and that he needed to talk to my boss, Ken. I was in a bad marriage, but married was married, and this guy was too perfect. He came back when Ken was there, but Ken kept telling him that I was the database expert and the only one who could give him an account on the system. It was hopeless. I was stuck working with him and trying to stifle this strong, persistent emotion. Zulfi remembers those days as, "I just figured you didn't like me or you had something going on in your life that made you crabby." Indeed.

Somewhere in the middle of the year that Zulfi and I worked together, I became pregnant with Ryan. I know that it is a bad idea to get pregnant to save a marriage, but I think that is what I did unconsciously. Zulfi was still finishing his degree, so we continued working together. I eventually accepted that we could be friends and coworkers without my having to be nasty to him in order to keep my distance.

Zulfi took a consulting job that meant he traveled about 95 percent of the time. He later shared that it was hard for him to be around me, too, wanting more than friendship and knowing I was married. He also shared that he did not date much because he was hoping that I would figure out that I could leave my marriage.

I finally divorced Larry in 1993, after three tumultuous years of trying to make things work, getting my two half brothers through school, and navigating Ryan's often draining medical and developmental issues. I began saying after those three years that I no longer believed in Hell. Whatever I may have done or would possibly do in the future, I am quite sure I have paid for it. I do know that is up to God, but it is certainly how I felt about those three years.

That year, 1993, was a big one for us. Ryan started preschool, and I started graduate school. The next two years would be as happy and peaceful as the previous three had been anguishing and difficult. Larry and I agreed that Ryan and I would stay in our house, and he would rent an apartment. It was a gracious gesture on his part. Our relationship has improved over time, and I am grateful that he continues to help support Ryan.

Zulfi and I had stayed in touch throughout those crazy three years and started dating in 1994. We were married in August of 1995. Ryan was so happy. Normally, he did not like to dress up, but he adored his little white   edo because I told him he would wear it "when we marry Buddy." When the day came, Ryan and I walked down the aisle together to begin our new life with Buddy.

Since marriage is hard even when it's good, Zulfi and I decided to go on a Retrouvaille marriage retreat in 2014. The retreat was in Indianapolis, just far enough away to seem like a getaway, but not too far to worry much about our kids, who were in the hands of our great OT caregivers.

During the retreat, I shared with Zulfi how puzzling it is to me that people are surprised at how much he loves Ryan. He agreed that it was puzzling to him, too. He did say that most men tell him they would have a hard time raising someone else's child, especially if handicapped. He found that sad, too. Then he shared how he feels about Ryan, and I simply cried and fell in love more deeply than I already was. He said, "Ryan is so easy to love. His love is unconditional, and he is so pure. I feel so fortunate to have (you and) Ryan to love. For me, it would not be a travesty in life not to *be* loved; it would be a travesty to not have someone *to love*."

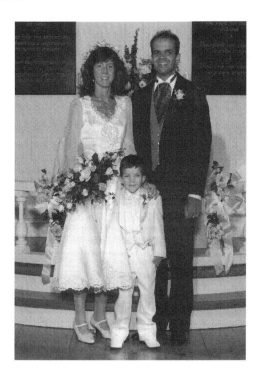

4

Cast of Characters

"It takes a village to raise a child."
– African proverb.

Some of the Wonderful People in Ryan's Life

Acknowledgments typically go in the very front or very back of books. Since I am pretty non-typical (I suppose the correct word is atypical), I am putting them here because no book about Ryan would be complete without acknowledging some of the many wonderful people who make or have made his life and our lives easier and better. There are stories about people in our lives elsewhere in the book. These acknowledgments, rather descriptions and stories, are here not just because I want to acknowledge or thank these wonderful people; I certainly hope that I have done that in person and/or by cards or letters, often. The descriptions and stories about the people in our lives are here primarily in order to share information that might be useful to the reader. For example, it is my hope that by describing what was most helpful about a caregiver or health care provider, that the reader will be equipped to know what to ask for should the need arise. Of course, if these wonderful people feel acknowledged and blessed, that is OK, too. Any list, even a long one, of acknowledgments runs the risk of leaving out someone important. That is certainly not the intention.

Most of the names and stories have been changed. Sometimes because I could not reach the person to obtain permission, sometimes because the name is not important, such as when the description represents all such caregivers being described. Sometimes because the person did not want to be named. If the person is named, I obtained permission in writing to use his or her name.

If medical professionals are true healers, and I have good stories, I may have used their real names if I obtained permission. If we had a less than positive experience, I have changed their names or left them nameless. In that case, I have also changed the story a bit so that it will not be recognizable or have left them out of the book altogether. The goal here is not to hurt, but to help make other people's journeys better by sharing some of the pain and joy.

They are in no particular order, which is to say, the order that I thought of them, and then I tried to re-order them in some kind of mostly chronological order, definitely *not* any sort of ranking.

Some of the first helpers were Ryan's godparents, the Hillyards, and their family. His godmother babysat three days a week so that I could continue my job. I did not want to return to work and was resentful that Larry "made" me. I was willing to make the necessary adjustments so that we did not need my salary. Larry was not. As with everything, I made the best of it and saw the silver lining. The silver lining at that time was the **Hillyard family.**

If it had not been for their help, I might have gone crazy. They loved Ryan like their own and saw him as the pure soul that he is. As one of many, many examples of their love and help: there was one time when Larry was out of town and I felt overwhelmed with Ryan's care, especially not being able to run, which made everything better for me. Knowing that they were all studying to be doctors or nurses and that I would be in a loving environment, I asked if I could bring Ryan and spend the night at their house. It was uncharacteristic of me to need and ask for such help and was just one of many lessons I would learn from Ryan. I am eternally grateful to them for being there.

Trudy was Ryan's first teacher at Park Special School. She was a real gem. It was she who pointed out how often I called Ryan "my buddy" by letting me know that when anyone asked Ryan his name, he answered "Buddy." I recall that my brother, George, used to call his son, Kevin, "my little buddy," too. I suppose it is a term of endearment in our family. Later, Ryan called my brother, Kenny, Buddy. Soon after we became close to Zulfi, Ryan called him Buddy, and he became "the Buddy" ever after.

Jackie was Ryan's second teacher. Ryan (and I) loved her so much that he had a very bad year after she stopped being his teacher. The next teacher was Ruth, whom, after that first difficult year, Ryan grew to love in later years. For many years, Ryan had Jackie's husband Dennis, who was the most beloved of all his teachers. Dennis had the perfect mix of patience and tough love for Ryan, and he soared under his guidance. With a lot of transition help from Dennis, Ryan had a couple of very good years with Tracy, another teacher Ryan loved a great deal.

We have a lovely picture of **Jackie, Dennis, and Tracy** hugging Ryan in the church after his First Communion. The frame was given to Ryan by my friend and one of his biggest fans, another Tracy.

Dr. Marsha Patay. There are not enough good adjectives for "Dr. Marsha." I have come to distrust many Western Medical Doctors and have become disgusted with their arrogance, the staff who protect them as gods and who treat patients as second-class folks who have nothing better to do than wait for hours in their uncomfortable waiting rooms after rushing to get there on time.

Our journey with doctors could fill another book, but I will just say here that Dr. Marsha is an *exception*. She treated me as an equal, as someone who is intelligent and knew things that she needed to know in order to care for Ryan. She trusted my intuition and respected my wishes. I had the same trust for her. The one time when we had a mix up on medicine, she and I were able to get through a difficult discussion and have a stronger relationship because of it.

She was warm and loving and knew Ryan inside and out. As a new physician (he was among her first patients), she was complemented by the white-haired Dr. Aslan for catching Ryan's problems before anyone else. She truly did stand out as a brilliant healer, which is very high praise from me.

Once, when we had to call the office while she was on maternity leave, I insisted that the doctor on call consult with her at home. After much resistance, the office manager *allowed* the doctor to call her. (What does *that* statement say about the state of Western pediatric offices?) The doctor later acknowledged, "I know now why you insisted I call her — I had Ryan's chart in my hand, and *she was 'reading' it to me.*"

Perhaps she was not able to be this way for all of her patients. I do not know. I do know that she saved Ryan's life at least three times. I am eternally grateful to her. I cried the day I got her letter announcing her early retirement to be able to spend more time with her own children. I was happy for her and them, but very worried for us.

Dr. Inez Hung is perhaps the reason I was not depressed about Dr. Marsha's retirement for long. She is very, very special, too, and we looked forward to forming a close relationship with her. She and Dr. Marsha told me that it is OK for me to ask Dr. Inez to call her. Knowing that made me feel a lot better. Somehow, I doubted I would have to call.

Dr. Jorge Sergio is retired now, but was the founder of the practice that Dr. Marsha was and Dr. Inez still is in. He is another rare gem. I will never forget two events that best illustrate how special he is.

When he picked Ryan up for the first time, it was as though he was the only child in the universe, and I was no longer in the room. There was some sort of magic going back and forth between his hands and Ryan's warm, soft body. Ryan smiled and he smiled back, a pure soul to a pure healer.

The other time was one morning when, as usual, I was rushing to work, doing several things at once in order to get out the door, and I needed to call for an appointment for Ryan. I noticed as I was dialing that it was five minutes to 8:00, so I started to hang up. I knew the office staff would not pick up the phone at five minutes *before* 8:00; they rarely even picked it up at five minutes *after* 8:00. Before I could hang up, I heard, "Jorge Sergio here." I said quickly, "Oh, sorry, Dr. Sergio, I need to make an appointment; I'll call back in a few minutes." He sounded almost hurt, "I know how to do that." I smiled. He made the appointment as though it was the most important thing he had to do that day. What a guy. It was moments like that that restored my faith, not just in doctors, but also in life.

Dr. Kadri Aslan is one of my very few heroes. If you close your eyes and imagine the stereotypical "mad scientist" with a shock of white hair, except instead of "mad," give him a kind, peaceful, and friendly face, you have the image of Dr. Aslan.

Dr. Aslan is an exception to Western medicine, perhaps because he is not Western. I guess it is not a fair comparison, but he is here, and I am very glad we crossed paths.

The two things Dr. Aslan did that make him special to me (besides being a brilliant geneticist) are:

Refusing to tell Ryan's paternal grandmother that she was the reason her son, Larry, Ryan's biological father, is a carrier and hence the reason Ryan has this rare disorder. Human eggs apparently have a "shelf life." And for some reason, when a woman has her first child later in life, the risk for chromosome abnormalities goes way up. One of the many things I learned doing research on DNA was that at age 35 the curve for chromosome disorders turns exponential.

I always respected Dr. Aslan's not telling her the reason for the balanced condition in Larry and, subsequently, the unbalanced condition in Ryan, even when Ryan's paternal grandparents were blaming me (my jogging during pregnancy) for Ryan's health problems.

His reasoning was simple. "... no good can come of it. She will not be having any more children and will only feel bad."

The other event that made him exceptional to me was the day I went to see him and our neurologist Dr. Burris:

I had just finished months of research on Ryan's chromosome disorder — the sort of research where you run into brick walls at every turn. For example, partial trisomy 12 was not even listed in the National Organization of Rare Diseases. There are about 12 cases in "the medical literature," and none of them is exactly Ryan's chromosome configuration.

I tracked down the resident geneticist who too-excitedly found information on Ryan's disorder when Ryan was three weeks old and in one of our local children's hospitals for pyloric stenosis. I enlisted the help of the research librarian at Washington University Medical School

Library to find all the known cases of trisomy 12, partial or not. I printed everything that I could from the internet on meiosis, the genome project and chromosome disorders. I did the same for the brain and seizure disorders. I had a list of 40 questions. After weeks of digging, I narrowed my list to about 25, split them into two categories, brain and genes, and made "consultation appointments" with Dr. Burris, our wonderful neurologist, and Dr. Aslan, the kind geneticist who diagnosed Ryan's disorder.

Now each of these "specialists" charges about $300 for a twenty-minute visit. I personally think they deserve it; I am not begrudging them, just noting the cost.

After spending about an hour and a half with me, patiently fielding my questions and answering them in a manner that any intelligent, educated, but non-geneticist, person could understand, Dr. Aslan asked me to keep him posted on Ryan's condition every few years. As we shook hands goodbye, he paid me a high compliment, "I wish all my patients' parents were like you."

I dreaded getting that bill, which I knew insurance would not cover because I was just a mom asking questions, after all.

Weeks went by. Finally, so that I would not be surprised with a bill when I could not pay it, I decided to call Dr. Aslan's office. When I inquired about the bill, his equally kind office manager said, "Dr. Aslan said there would be no charge. He enjoyed your visit very much." Wow.

Dr. Garret Burris, our beloved neurologist. Dr. Burris was the unlucky recipient of a very frustrated and disillusioned family trying desperately to care for a child who started having seizures after a bad fall while at a party with his father. We were dealing with the anger of that on top of the unpredictable and scary seizures.

We came to Dr. Burris after leaving the practice of "the best neurologist in St. Louis, if not the country." I am certain that is a true statement in many senses. I liked him very much. He was warm and had a good "bedside manner." I especially liked his associate. However, this neurologist saw patients on Mondays from 9 am to 11 am. We had to arrive at least 15 minutes early for our 9 am appointment. We moved heaven and earth to get there on time and finally got to see him at 10:55 a.m.! That simply did not work in our life. I will not dwell on the fact that his office staff was rude and lost Ryan's chart at a time when it nearly made the difference between life and death. We left this doctor's practice and prayed that Dr. Burris would be better.

That doctor, our former neurologist, was also a friend of Dr. Burris; so, needless to say, we did not get started on the best foot. To his credit, Dr. Burris was patient with us, and we now have a very good working relationship. He gave Ryan and us very good care during our time with him. He has since moved on to teach and practice in semi-retirement. We made our last appointment to say goodbye, and he said he would pass us on to a younger doctor in his practice. I am very grateful.

Dr. Burris saw us through a tough couple of years, where we were in his office and/or the ER more than we were anywhere else, or at least it seemed that way.

I will never forget the day our baby, Lauren, who had no known medical reason to have seizures, had a febrile (fever-induced) seizure. I was uncharacteristically hysterical. I wanted to scream, "Wrong child; different father! Why her? Why me? Why us?" I think I actually did scream those phrases at someone, likely my sweet husband Zulfi.

During that time, Dr. Burris was more a doctor to *me* than to Lauren. He understood what I was feeling, and he articulated it and was reassuring. He said, "She will probably have another seizure in 24 hours." In exactly 25 hours, he called back to check, which was then Sunday morning. Lauren had just finished her seizure, and Dr. Burris talked me down from the ledge. Words cannot adequately articulate how grateful I felt for his kindness and care.

Another special thing about Dr. Burris is that he personally escorted his patients back to his office. In addition, I have never had to wait more than 15 minutes to see him or more than 30 minutes for him to return a call. I am so grateful for him and his nurse, Val, who was a great extension of Dr. Burris and the other doctors in the practice.

It is not just the doctors who are the healers. In fact, it seems that we have been blessed with many special nurses, OT's (occupational therapists), and PT's (physical therapists).

One of the most special nurses in our life was **Heidi Pelant Gioi**a, our OB/GYN nurse practitioner. She was there the day after Ryan was born, and even though she is *my* nurse, the way she has taken care of me has helped me take care of Ryan. She takes time to talk to her patients, works with an individual's ability (or inability) to pay, truly cares, and responds as quickly as possible. I think she probably has the same view of rules as I do, "Obey all rules that make sense or for which the consequences for not doing so are too great," and "sometimes it's easier to get forgiveness than permission." She is a real gem, and I was able to be a better mother to Ryan because of her excellent care for over 30 years.

I love this quote from the movie *Fried Green Tomatoes*, "It's a well known fact that there are angels on earth masqueradin' as humans." **Jeanne Kloeckner**, OTD and friend, is one of them. We met through our daughters' preschool, and the connection was instant. Jeanne is one of those rare people who exudes peace. I was instantly attracted to her soul and am glad that we remain friends even though we have both "graduated" from the preschool where our girls went.

She has given Ryan and me many gifts, including recommending Sue Hofmann, a physical therapist and lifeline, and providing needed cranial sacral therapy on Ryan, as well as the rest of us.

One day, unbeknownst to her, she invited me to tea during a time when I may have "lost it" otherwise. She was dealing with her own family issues and could not have known what a blessing just being in her peaceful presence was for me. Somehow I think she did know.

Sue Hofmann, PT. Sue is someone who is very easy to talk to. She is such a good listener, a natural healer, and such a caring health professional that there always seems just one more thing to say. She came into our lives when I was extremely frustrated with the answers I was getting from physical therapy at school, from the orthopedist, from the orthotists, and the lab that made Ryan's braces.

We scheduled a one-hour visit, and she left four hours later, confirming everything I had been saying for the last three years about what was going on with Ryan.

She now accompanies me on visits and does everything from calling doctors for me and finding deals on used equipment to listening to me share and complain about how unfair life is sometimes.

She should be paid four times what she charges, but she usually does not bill us for half of the hours she works anyway. Thank you, God, for Sue.

Mike, the Orthotist. Mike is a very special health provider, too. He has made Ryan's braces for many years. Like me, he does just about everything Sue asks him to do, trusting her as knowing what Ryan needs. And occasionally, when he suggests something different, it is for a good reason. They work well together so Ryan can walk as well as possible.

Thicker than Water

George, known as FOB (favorite *older* brother — because we should not have favorite siblings or favorite children), is also known as my hero. Sadly, there are few heroes in the world. Ryan's Uncle George is one. He is a good husband to Aunt **Sherri**, a great father to Kevin and Shaunna, a strong, faithful servant of God, and a hard worker. I am very happy that we have grown closer once again, and everyone comes to visit every other Christmas. All of Ryan's uncles make a point of taking Ryan driving (his favorite thing) and making sure he is happy.

Kenny is my brother and the first Buddy. There are so many stories. The two that come to mind are how Kenny lovingly let Ryan ride on his shoulder while we walked all over town. I do not even remember where we were or why, but we had been walking for a long while. Kenny seemed so happy holding Ryan, and Ryan was happy holding onto him.

The other story also involves holding. Again, I do not recall the details, but Ryan was in the hospital *again*. They were doing tests to try to find out why he was having so many seizures. They had to give him anesthesia so he would keep the probes on his head for the test, and it knocked him out. It was hard for all of us to watch him being poked and prodded. One particularly clueless anesthetist looked at me in exasperation after trying to put probes on Ryan before sedation, and said, "Can't you tell him to be still?!" Sure. I will get right on that.

Actually, I got right on walking quietly out of the room and asking for a different anesthesiology tech.

Another beautiful memory of my brother and Ryan was made during a particularly difficult morning. Ryan had essentially passed out from exhaustion, and Kenny said, "I'll hold him so you can have a break. Go get something to eat." We left for a short while to get something to eat. When we came back, Ryan was still resting peacefully in Kenny's arms. We sat down and talked. I offered several times to take Ryan from him, but he was worried Ryan would wake up. He held Ryan for nearly six hours, allowing Ryan to get some much-needed sleep. All these years later, I still remember the look on Kenny's face as he held Ryan and the peaceful way that Ryan slept in his arms. I always knew he would make a good father. I am so glad God blessed him with his wife **Mistie**, and their daughter, Brooke, many years later.

"Uncle Steben" and **Uncle Brian** lived with us from the time Ryan was two months old until age three. Steven still calls Ryan "Pip Squeak." We have many happy memories of Ryan with Uncle Steven, and it is sad that he lives so far away that we rarely see him.

Fortunately, we get to see **Brian**, his wife **Allison**, and their children, every year or so. All of Ryan's uncles, when they visit, take him for car or truck rides, one of his favorite things.

Ryan loves to hear **Papa** (my Uncle Tony) whistle, and Papa loves to whistle for Ryan. He also takes Ryan for car rides when we visit him and **Gigi** (Aunt Trisha) or they come here. Ryan is also close to Papa and Gigi's daughter **Aunt Janet**, who is like my sister. She cooks for us when she comes. Janet's daughter, **Amanda**, came to visit when Kiran was born. She helped take care of all of us, even though she was very young at the time.

Easily one of Ryan's favorite people on the planet, "Uncle Moke" (**Uncle Mark**) used to take Ryan to speech lessons twice a week and still takes him to dinner twice a week since speech stopped. He makes Ryan laugh, and laughter is such an important key to happiness.

You know the saying, "Someone always has it worse." I hate that. Truly. I want to say, "Yeah, and someone always has it *better*, too, and right now what I am going through is hard, can't you just hear that?"

My friend, **Laura**, has endured so much and probably "has it worse" than anyone I know well, but she is one of those wonderful, rare people who would never say that. I have told many people "I am the happiest person I know," and she is also one of the happiest people I know. We both have many, many reasons to be happy, but also both have more reasons than most folks have to be sad. We both choose happiness at least most days. That is most likely the biggest reason that we connected instantly at work and have remained friends for over 20 years.

Most people think that Laura and I look alike, that we could be sisters. For a while when we worked together, and our hair was cut and styled similarly, some folks thought we were twins.

One of our favorite stories is about being "sisters." We were changing into our running clothes after work, when someone we barely knew came in to say, "We have a bet going; we know you're sisters, but some of us think you are twins." Without even batting an eye, I responded, "Yes, we're twins." Laura did not correct me, but after the woman left said, "You are so funny. Why did you say that?" "Because we have twin souls and twin hearts, and most of the time, twin brains." She just hugged me.

We laid the foundation of our friendship during those runs. Three times a week, we treated ourselves to running after work and shared stories. One of the most vivid and happy memories we both have is the night we ran around Washington University Medical School's campus in circles because it was dark and not safe in the nearby park for two women to run alone. It was five degrees Fahrenheit, which was bad enough. We were also being pelted with freezing rain. I do not think Laura had gloves on. While we ran, she told me the whole story about her son, Danny; how he went from a vibrant five-year-old to the silent, low-functioning person he is now — the sad result of medical care for a brain tumor gone wrong.

I was crying the whole time. While I was honored to be the recipient of the intimate details of the story, I was so sad that my good friend had lost her son. I was deeply feeling the pain of this beautiful lady. I knew we would be close forever, and we have been.

We branched out from our pour-your-heart-out runs one weekend to a hotel seminar/retreat for which she had registered. She invited Ryan and me to come during the evening break to swim in the pool and talk. Ryan was two, I think, and still not walking independently. Danny was in a wheelchair, her daughter Jenny, who is Ryan's age, was running all over, and her last child, David, was still a baby. We must have looked quite the group: David on Laura's hip, her pushing Danny's wheelchair with one hand, me holding Jenny's hand (or running after her) while navigating Ryan with his walker. It remains one of our happiest memories during the time our friendship was blossoming.

Ryan's sister, Lauren, is named for "Aunt Laura." I could not find an Indian name I could pronounce, and I wanted to give her a special name.

I changed it to Lauren to be a little different. I suppose I knew, somehow, that Lauren would be different in a very special way.

During the short period Ryan and Kiran needed to be at a daycare, we met a special employee we later called **Muppet**. One day, Muppet noticed Ryan wasn't himself. She made a point of holding his hand most of the day to ease his emotional discomfort. Because of this level of care, I talked to her about working for us. We arranged care that would work with her and my college schedules. She took care of all three children for many years. She was like family.

Her Name is "Kadie"

If you ask Ryan about someone and he cannot think of her name, he will usually say "Kadie," his way of pronouncing Katie. I think that is because we have had so many special Katies in our life — babysitters, nurses, teachers, assistants, speech therapists, and other caregivers. It is a popular name, especially in this big Catholic town of St. Louis. No book about Ryan's journey would be complete without expressing gratitude for all of our Katies, even the ones Ryan called Katie who had different names. This is in gratitude for all the "Kadies" past, present and future. You know who you are. To name just a few ...

Katie, the wife of a friend of Zulfi's, quickly became my friend. She is a nurse and a great mom. One day, I found her sitting with Ryan on the grass in the front lawn taking a break from a birthday party. They were having a great time. She and her family have since moved away, but we keep in touch on social media. Some people touch your life ever so slightly, but so deeply that they stay in your heart forever. This Katie is an angel who represents all the special people in our lives.

Kadie is one of Ryan's favorite people. The spelling of her name is great because that is how Ryan pronounces all versions of Katie. She is the daughter of a friend I used to work with and was the babysitter of choice for years.

"Marrory" (**Mallory**) was never called Kadie, but was just as beloved. Mallory was the first of the Washington University OT students to care for Ryan. She set the care bar high, and, thankfully, all of the students who have come after her have met or exceeded it. She also made him a soft Woody blanket that he loves.

Kari is an angel among us. Kari was the second Washington University student to come. Ryan still asks for Kari even though she has not been a direct part of our lives for a few years.

Chris works with AADD (Association on Aging with Developmental Disabilities). While he was never called Kadie, he is the male version of one of these beautiful (inside and out) ladies.

As I re-read this section, I realized that the stories I could write could fill an entire book. I could not and would not be where I am today without all the special people in our lives. I am so afraid and quite certain that I have left some out.

Thank You Letters

Your kindness should be known to all.
– Philippians 4:5
http://www.usccb.org/bible

Taking Time

For as long as I can remember, I have tried to take time to say thank you for kindnesses and good service. It seems like the right thing to do, and I hope it balances out the times I have had to point out injustices or bad service. Unfortunately, many of these thank you letters have been in the form of handwritten cards, which the recipients have. I will include a representative sample here to illustrate how Ryan has taught me to walk in gratitude.

Take Me Out to the Ball Game

April 15, 2003

Mr. Base Ball (not his real name)
250 Stadium Plaza
St. Louis, MO 63102

Dear Mr. Ball,

My family would like to express our appreciation for the recent help of two of your ushers, Chrissy and Carl. They are usually the ushers for our section, 274, that we have shared as season ticket holders for the past 5 years.

They are always very friendly and helpful, but on April 5, they went above and beyond. Our handicapped son, Ryan, has recently gotten a wheelchair. Chrissy met me at the doorway, Carl offered to put the wheel chair away for us, and Chrissy helped me lead/carry Ryan up the steps to our seats. They retrieved the wheelchair a few minutes before the game was over so that we would not get trampled by the crowd.

They made the game more pleasant for Ryan, which made it fun for all of us. My kids love going to the "ball game." I'm sure a big part of this is your helpful, friendly staff. I just wanted you to know how helpful they were and how very much we appreciated it.

The Jeevanjees: Zulfi, Theresa, Ryan, Kiran and Lauren

Just a few of the people to whom I have written handwritten cards in order to say thanks through the years …
Jeanne Kloeckner, OTD; Susan Hofmann, PT; Dr. Marsha; Dr. Enrico Stazzone; the whole of Southview Special School; Dennis and Jackie Ball; Tracy Wolz; Kathy and all of Sarah Care; nurses and aides at

St. Louis Children's Hospital; St. Luke's Hospital; Cardinal Glennon Children's Hospital; and the ambulance crew in South County.

An email thank you note and another miracle ...

From: Theresa Jeevanjee, Ph.D.
Sent: Wednesday, December 03, 2003
To: Annette
Subject: Angels
Dear Annette,
cc: Mikey

I just wanted to relay a story. Do you remember that at Teresa's wedding I lost the angel "coin" that Beth gave me? Tonight is the night that she died a year ago — it has been a very sad day for me for several reasons. But, it was also Kiran's first Reconciliation, so we were sitting in church, and I was happy to be lost in the beautiful music. I have a little container with Vaseline in it for chapped lips that I keep in my pocket. When I opened it tonight to use some, I found the angel! I have used it a dozen times since the wedding, and it is sealed. I cannot imagine how it could have gotten in there. Either I missed it, or some miracle put the angel there. Either way, I found the angel and got the warmest feeling that Beth was sending a message. My father died the day after Thanksgiving. As you know George, Kenny and I went to visit him right before Teresa's wedding — a week before he died, so at least I got to see him before he died. We are all going to the funeral on Friday. He will get the full military honors (21 gun salute etc.) because he was an honored, wounded Veteran. That would have made him happy. Please keep us in your prayers. I really enjoyed seeing you and Doug. Take good care.

Mikey, we miss you. Kiran wants you to be at her First Communion. She was kind of upset you weren't here tonight (I told her that we didn't even ask since kids don't really "bring their own priests to Reconciliation," so she was ok as long as you come in May. I'll keep you posted for the date.) We are not going to have our Christmas party this year because Ryan is having surgery on December 15 to help his walking. But, maybe you, Annette and Doug could come to dinner while my aunt is here (December 13 onward).

Much love and gratitude,
Theresa

From: Mike May, S.J.
Sent: Saturday, December 06, 2003 11:23 PM
To: Theresa Jeevanjee
Re: Angels
Theresa,

Whether it is a miracle or a magic trick, I like the story. I also chuckled at the idea of being brought to a first reconciliation. Let me know when the date will be for the first communion. I would not have been available for the reconciliation since I was in Houston for my brother's funeral. He died the Sunday before Thanksgiving. He was 48, but had been in bad health. The emotions are tangled since that is too young to die, but he had also suffered enough for us to be ready to let go. There is no easy way to bury a close relative, no matter what the previous story was. Keep me in your prayers. I am keeping you and yours in mine.

Mikey

Theresa L. Jeevanjee
St. Louis, MO 63129

December 22, 1997

Southview Transportation
To Whom It May Concern:

I am writing this to express my appreciation for our new bus driver, Perry, and assistant, Peggy. They are two of the nicest people I have ever met. They are also the best team we have had since my son, Ryan Maxwell, started riding route 52 in 1993.

People who are happy doing their jobs seem few and far between these days. I thought it would be worthwhile to take the time to let you know how much we appreciate seeing their smiling faces every morning and afternoon.

They seem to go the extra step, too. My son has been behaving badly occasionally on the bus. Instead of getting irritated, as many would do, they are working with me to find solutions to the problem. They are very encouraging when Ryan behaves well.

Ryan can't wait to get on the bus every morning. He greets them with a very enthusiastic hello and "high five" — something he did not do in the past. I hope they continue to be our bus team as long as Ryan goes to Southview.

Thank you very much,
Theresa L. Jeevanjee

August 12, 2004

To Ryan's PT and Teacher at the time (and other Southview staff),

I hope you have had a great summer. Ryan's casts are off! They came off August 3. He has done very well so far. He sleeps well about half the nights and tolerates his night braces (new immobilizers) fairly well.

The braces are locked, and we have not yet released them to allow him to bend his knee while walking. We are taking this one day at a time, so there will not be written instructions from Dr. Stazzone for a while. For now, please allow "walking" and standing in his braces as tolerated. (Dr. Stazzone said, if Ryan says to stop, then we should stop.) He can walk with his walker or holding hands. We have had success having him hold onto our shoulders and walk behind us. This helps him to stand straighter.

As always you have my permission to talk to any of Ryan's caregivers about his treatment or care. I will be out of town from August 13 to August 19. You may leave a message on my cell phone and I will call you back if you need to talk to me. I look forward to hearing your input about this. Thanks for all you have done, Carrie, to help Ryan.

Here are some important numbers so that you don't have to look them up. (Numbers removed for this publication.)

Talk to you soon,

Ryan's mom

Theresa L. Jeevanjee
St. Louis, MO 63129

September 25, 1998

St. Louis Children's Hospital
Same-Day Surgery Center
Dear Same-Day Surgery Staff:

Please accept this letter as a small token of our sincere appreciation for taking such good care of our son, Ryan Maxwell, today. Everyone we encountered was not only pleasant and helpful, but seemed happy to "go the extra step" when Ryan needed special care.

I would especially like to thank Ms. Wellington for her warmth and professionalism. From the time she first called us to preregister us until we left, she was kind and helpful. It is so rare these days to find administrative staff who do their jobs well, even more rare to find them that smile while they do it, and simply amazing that she is able to be that way at 6:30 in the morning! You are fortunate to have Ms. Wellington working for you.

We would also like to thank Dr. Luke and his nurse, Cindy, for their efforts in coordinating the tube surgery with Dr. Sommer's dental work. In addition to being excellent medical professionals, you both have a gift for working with children *and their parents.* We are grateful Dr. Luke was the ENT (Ear Nose and Throat) specialist on call when we first brought Ryan to the CARES unit at Children's.

We are also grateful to have such superb anesthesia doctors, Dr. Underhill and Dr. Roberts. Dr. Underhill allowed me to carry Ryan into the operating room (O.R.) so that he wasn't so scared and made us feel very comfortable about the whole procedure. Dr. Roberts was very good with Ryan, took time to answer our questions, and made us feel at ease.

All the doctors and nurses we saw were wonderful. Dr. Jem was very professional, and we were impressed by the fact that the O.R. nurse, Ms. Dean, introduced herself to us and asked if we had any questions. The recovery room nurse, Ms. Smith, was especially kind to Ryan even while he was being very difficult about his IV (intravenous tube). She offered me options to make Ryan more comfortable and made me feel like I was a valued participant in my son's care.

Finally, I would like to add that the person who did the most to make our stay easier was our nurse, Sherry. Ryan has Partial Trisomy 12, a rare chromosome disorder, which includes global developmental delay. He does not like to be touched or have anything attached to his body. Sherry never showed signs of being impatient or bothered by any of Ryan's struggles. If Ryan fought her about something she was doing, she just came up with an alternative method of doing it — sometimes two or three alternative methods!

Ms. Meyer is a special person and an exceptional nurse. We are grateful for the attentive care that she gave to all of us.

Thanks again to all of you for doing so many things right, you have hit upon the formula for working as a team to make same-day surgery as painless as possible — from the way you keep parents informed down to refreshments in the waiting room.

(Names were changed because individuals could not be contacted for permission. The letter is included to share traits of good caregivers.)

Sincerely,

Theresa L. Jeevanjee

February 2002

Dear Kenny,

Hi. It was lovely talking to you. I thought I was doing fine, but right when I sat down to dinner, I started crying and could hardly eat. I guess it will hit me in stages. I'm glad you are going to the "funeral." I need to go and going with you will be easier.

I'm calling to ask you a favor. There's a long history to this, which I will save for a phone call, but I thought I should give you some advance warning.

I just found out that Aunt Trish will be in Portugal on Grandparent's Day. Grandparent's Day is a super big deal at Kiran's and Lauren's school. Unfortunately, I did not know what a big deal it was until the day OF the event last year. Kiran and I parted in tears that day – she missing the Grandmother she has never known; me missing the mother we lost too soon. I vowed never to be caught off guard again.

I have spoken to the Head of School about the lack of communication about this day, and he apologized and since then has publicized the event well in advance. We already know the date: March 5. They are allowed to bring a Grandparent, other relative, or "special friend."

When I told Kiran that Gigi would be in Portugal, she announced, "Uncle Kenny will come." No pressure. I told her that you certainly would come if you could, but that you might be working or any number of things. She said I would do if you cannot come. I think I am going to plan to come even if you can.

So, please mark your calendar – and if it's not too much trouble, please come. It's an early morning event where you would escort your nieces to a reception and an assembly. I think the whole thing is over by 10:30. I certainly will understand if you cannot come, but I thought I would ask.

I would love to see a happy face on that little girl I left crying a year ago. It kind of bugs me that they do this, but given that they do, I would rather have her happy than sad.

Thanks for considering it.

Much love,

Teri

(Uncle Kenny drove all night to make it. He spent Grandparents Day with a very happy Kiran and the evening with a very happy Ryan. Kiran and I sent a follow-up thank you note, which I could not find.)

Theresa L. Jeevanjee
St. Louis, MO 63129

September 25, 1998

Dr. Harold Sommer
St. Louis, MO

Dear Dr. Sommer,

Please accept this letter as a small token of my appreciation for all the things you and your nurse, Jan, did to make my son, Ryan Maxwell, feel more comfortable about his dental work done today.

Jan worked very hard coordinating the dental work with Dr. Luke's office so that you could do the dental work while Ryan was already under anesthesia for tube surgery. She kept me informed and gave me important information about insurance coverage. I am very grateful for her friendly help.

I have always been impressed by your office, not just by your warm, professional staff, but because it is such a fun and comfortable place for kids. You somehow managed to bring all that with you when you came to the Same-Day Surgery Center today to do the work. Ryan was very excited to see you, and you made us feel comfortable about the procedure. We are so grateful for you and the caring way you do your job!

And, thank you for the balloons with the "goodie bag" attached. What a sweet, thoughtful thing to do. Ryan loves Mickey Mouse and balloons, so he got a double treat.

We look forward to seeing you at our next visit.

Sincerely,

Theresa L. Jeevanjee

Ryan turned 22 April 11, which is 18 years older than his predicted lifespan of four. We have had quite the journey. We have retired two pediatricians, have gone through six physical therapists and likely as many neurologists. We finally found a neurologist who would Listen, and today we had to say goodbye to him. He got a great opportunity to "slow down" and to teach other doctors while directing the children's neurology clinic associated with Baylor.

We made an appointment to say goodbye and then later sent this note:

Dear Dr. Burris,

Attached is the picture I took of you and Ryan today. Thank you for making this journey easier for me, for being patient in the beginning when we were tired beyond all coping and the last thing we needed was for Ryan to have seizures, thank you for valuing my opinion, and for caring for my son. As you know, having a son like Ryan with a rare chromosome disorder (one of twelve in the medical literature), we have tested the medical system to its breaking. I have always been grateful for you and have sent many patients to you (not sure you even knew that).

As I told you today, the thing that makes it easier for me to let go of you is knowing that you will be helping future doctors. That is even more important than continuing to help kids.

Many blessings to you and your wife and the rest of your family as you embark on the next stage of your career. I will be praying daily for a long, happy life for you all.

In deep gratitude,

Theresa (Ryan's mom)

Dear Ryan,

While this at first reading is more about me than you, it is here along with its reply to illustrate how hard work and dedication can pay off. And saying thank you can make all the difference. You taught me that.

In gratitude,

Your mom

———————

Subject: thanks

Dear Ms. Norma,

I'm not sure how many years ago it was that I took my first ballet class at COCA, feeling like a cow in a fish bowl or a giraffe on roller skates. I think I was 42, so about 9 years ago. I started, I quit. I started again. Finally a few years ago, I decided that I needed more than once a week if I were going to stick with it. Throughout the journey you have been there, patiently putting up with me, who had to have been your worst student ever. I don't have your talent, but I do share your love of ballet. And I do benefit greatly from the physical and mental exercise and the camaraderie. Thanks for putting up with me all these years.

After we left our old studio, we started taking classes at Dance Center of Kirkwood for additional classes to COCA. They have an adult class that has every age from 30 to 82! Many of us danced in the Saturday performance. For me, it was my very first recital ever, at the age of 51! It was so much fun, and a dream come true for me.

We did Heliotrope Bouquet by Scott Joplin. As you probably know, Heliotrope is a purple flower, but the purple flowers on our costumes were an accident! Ms. Kathy picked the costume because it had long sleeves and some of the ladies prefer that. Serendipity.

Anyway, I just wanted to share a picture from the performance and to say thank you. There are many people at Dance Center who know you and recall what a great teacher you are. COCA has many great teachers, but no one has quite your way of explaining things. Thanks for sharing your gifts with me! Thanks for helping me do something that is hard for me, but that I love.

Gratefully,

Theresa Jeevanjee

Dear Theresa,

Thank you so much for the lovely letter and photo! You ladies look good!

To tell you the truth, when I saw that subject line "thanks," I was afraid you were saying "good-bye." I am so glad that is not the case. Your love definitely shows when you dance and that is why we all keep doing this.

See you in class!

Norma

The Thank-You Note I sent for Ryan's "See What Love Can Do" Party

Dear Friends,

I hope you will forgive me for writing one communal thank-you note. I want to thank each and every one of you for helping us make Ryan's birthday, graduation and "end of bus days" party so special. And if I took the time to write a hundred plus thank-you notes, it might be next year before you got it. Besides, in the happy chaos that surrounds a big party, presents got separated from cards, and I was very worried that I would mismatch the notes or miss something anyway. I also thought that sharing the story of the gifts might be nicer. I hope you agree.

After most people had gone from our happy celebration, our family and a few friends stayed and helped/watched Ryan open his presents, which is a special joy for us because for so many years, he would have nothing to do with presents. It was a nice consolation to him for having to get off the carriage. (You would think that five hours was long enough …☺)

I wish you could have seen his happy face as he opened each thoughtful card, lovingly read by Danielle, many containing gift cards and money. Some had offers for rides (one of his favorite things), some were attached to balloons — there were so many beautiful balloons that still fill our foyer and remind us of the happy party, some of those balloons ("badoons") were attached to stuffed animals, gummy bears, and cookies, one especially big cookie sandwich, which he has already happily devoured. So many of the cards had money, gift cards and donations to Fontbonne's Speech Clinic. Ryan got over $300 cash and more than that was donated to the clinic, one donation was $100! The presents (also happily opened) included a basketball (he loves to watch his sisters and mom play and to catch it once in a while), Woody towels, a book bag, two shirts and his caregiver, "Marrory," made him a soft and beautiful Woody blanket. There were stuffed animals, yard toys, pool toys, coloring kits, baseball games, a guardian angel medallion, lots of Oreos (his favorite cookie next to Mom's), picture frames, scrapbooks from beloved teachers, a Woody hat, two pair of sunglasses (he loves taking these off friends), books, cologne, a crystal candle stick holder, home-made canned beans, a Frisbee, chocolate, a hand-made card, and probably other things I've missed even though I tried to write them all down as Danielle, Dad and Buddy helped Ryan open gifts.

I think I counted 20 McDonald's gift cards ("Donald's money"), one for First Watch, six for Dewey's, one for Serendipity, one for Cold Stone Creamery, one for Yo My Goodness, one for Bread Company (Panera), two for Borders, one for Puddin' Head Books, two for Barnes and Noble, one for Steak and Shake, three for Target, two Visa Cards, and two wallets, one filled with money and a variety of gift cards. I took all of the restaurant gift cards and a good deal of cash and put it in the wallets (they don't quite close). Ryan and his Uncle Mark go out to eat once or twice to week (usually after Speech Clinic), and Ryan will enjoy "paying" at all his favorite places. I will use the other cards to buy him something he will enjoy. Kiran has already picked out books to share with the Borders cards. She goes to Puddin' Head Books and Barnes and Noble a lot and will get books there soon for Ryan.

I would also like to thank those who brought food and drinks. As most of you know, I love to cook and don't mind doing the whole meal/party. As time got closer and our garage fridge gave up, I realized I needed help. We've used Quizno's catering before with success, but when I got there the sign said it was closed for a week (REALLY?). In my quest for the next Quiznos, I found Crazy Bowls and Wraps — they deliver! Still slightly worried that I would not have enough food, I said yes to some folks who offered (which I don't usually do). People brought beautiful fruit sticks, cheese trays — some with mice (made out of a pear — clever), a lovely salad (which I did actually get to enjoy at 9 pm), several folks brought lovely wine (I'm keeping that ☺) and beer. One of my dear friends even brought me a present: dark chocolate, a tee shirt (from her mom on a recent trip) and a lovely tea towel.

During the party, many people offered to help. Several people washed dishes when we ran out and were always at hand for whatever I needed. One of my students helped get the two wheelchairs up the stairs so those young men could enjoy the party. I am grateful to each of you — it allowed me to enjoy the party without feeling stressed.

A very special thanks to Ryan's dad, Larry; the party was our (Mom, Buddy and Dad) gift to Ryan and for all his and Danielle's help. A very special thanks also to my husband, Saint Zulfikar, who not only puts up with my Irish rants (I am especially Irish the hour before the party starts), but he is responsible for the beautiful garden we enjoyed while eating, talking and waiting for the carriage. There would have been no party without him. And a deep, heartfelt thanks to Ryan's physical therapist, Saint Susan, (my "sister"), who provided all the grad decorations and stayed long after I collapsed in a heap and finished cleaning. I awoke the next morning expecting to finish cleaning, and Zulfi and Sue had washed every last dish and swept and mopped the kitchen floor. I don't think I've ever felt more loved.

I have not named everyone, and I have probably missed a gift or two, but Ryan hasn't. He was happier than I have ever seen him, and you helped make that happen. Thank you from the bottom of my heart. And thank you again for forgiving me for saving some time and sharing the "story of the presents" rather than sending over a hundred individual "thank you for the badoons for Ryan" type notes.

With love and gratitude,
Ryan's mom and family
Theresa, Zulfi ("Buddy"), Kiran, and Lauren

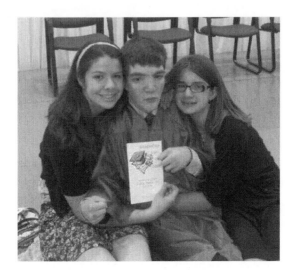

5

Advocating for Ryan

"I have told you this so that you might have peace in me.
In the world you will have trouble, but take courage,
I have conquered the world."
– John 16:33
http://www.usccb.org/bible

"I learned that courage was not the absence of fear,
but the triumph over it.
The brave man is not he who does not feel afraid,
but he who conquers that fear."
– Nelson Mandela

Advocacy

As I have mentioned before, the definition of "Advocate" is the "speaking or writing in favor of someone." It is what parents do for their children. I find it interesting that the word *advocat* in Latin and French also means lawyer. I have sometimes needed, but more often had to fight, lawyers in order to be Ryan's advocate. And I also find it interesting that I have often had to challenge doctors, who are supposed to be advocates for their patients. I have mentioned elsewhere the first time I stood up to be Ryan's advocate, here are some more stories.

Triage

January 13, 2004

"Thank you for that," I choked out as politely as I could manage while fighting back tears, and then I just hung up on Dr. Blasire (not his real name.)

"What an asshole," I thought, and I rarely swear. I suppose it is some consolation that I was right not to have him do Ryan's surgery. He embodies everything that is wrong with Western medicine. The visits with him when he would not even look at Ryan and kept saying, "kids with CP (cerebral palsy) ..." are still too fresh in my mind. Ryan does NOT have CP.

Ryan is just barely three weeks post-op from his hamstring and adductor lengthening surgeries (that are supposed to help him walk better), and we are almost as many nights without sleep. We have tried to take turns and even let Ryan stay with his father once to get a good night's sleep. Nevertheless, severe sleep deprivation is taking its toll. In fact, I am at the end of *everything*.

I do not have the energy to recount the whole of Ryan's surgery, much less the saga leading up to it. I suppose the tears after tonight's conversation represent the culmination of my frustration with all arrogant health professionals.

The fact that Ryan needed surgery at all is a result of arrogant health professionals in the first place. They were too busy, too smart, too important to listen to Ryan's mom. What does she know anyway — she "just" has a Ph.D., not an M.D.

The surgery itself went rather well. Dr. Sterling (not his real name) is a rare doctor: kind, patient, brilliant, and caring. One would have to have walked the journey with us to appreciate the depth of that compliment coming from me. He is a gift, and he gives freely of the many gifts he has been given fully.

The surgery was December 22, and I had 20-plus family members coming in spurts from December 13 through January 2 to help and visit. They were a great deal of help and support. More help and support than work, which I think is rare in families. I was and am very grateful.

Because one of my sisters-in-law is a nurse, Dr. Sterling was spared an emergency call during that time. Ryan had developed severe bedsores from his braces and adductor separator pillow. We did have to insist on a check up since our official post-op could not be scheduled until January 6. We were there for three hours. I was pleased that Dr. Sterling took the time to treat Ryan well.

Since then, we have been trying our best to be diligent with the equipment we have to help reinforce the surgery and all of the "attachments." These include a "stander," "soft braces," the adductor wedge with straps, and lots of bandages and cushions. Ryan has grown increasingly less tolerant of these things as he has healed and come off the pain medication and Valium.

For the last week, we have taken turns sleeping with him while he cries and fights to take off all the things attached to him. I have glued the Velcro to the adductor wedge so many times; it will not stick anymore. That having failed, we tried Ace bandages to keep the pillow attached to and separating his legs. He ripped it off. He usually collapses about 4 o'clock in the morning for a couple of hours. When 6:00 a.m.

rolls around, we have to get up and pretend we care about going about our days.

After a weekend of nearly no sleep, we resolved to call Dr. Sterling for "Plan B." We needed to know whether **not** using the adductor wedge would erase the effects of the surgery or not. If so, we needed some sleep medication that would not interfere with seizure meds, but would knock him out so that he would not notice the wedge.

Since Dr. Sterling is in surgery all day on Mondays, we decided it would be best to wait till Tuesday to call. There was no sense in trying to explain all this to someone else. Besides, we had already had two bad experiences with Dr. Blasire.

First thing Tuesday morning, I called their office. The operator always answers the phone with a cheery, "Where may I direct your call?" After weeks of frustration with trying to schedule the surgery in the first place, I felt like saying, "to any warm-blooded person, just not another voicemail that won't be checked until tomorrow." But I didn't; I politely said, "to Carla (not her real name), the triage nurse for Dr. Sterling, please."

As expected, Carla's voicemail picked up. I left a message for her to call and started to tackle the mountains of work on my desk. At least Carla returns her calls, which she did within ten minutes. I carefully relayed our frustration over the past few weeks and asked for either Dr. Sterling to call me back or for her to relay the message and let me know what to do. I reiterated that we needed either sleep medication or permission to leave off the braces so that Ryan could sleep. She seemed like she was carefully taking down the information and even asked for our pharmacy number.

Triage. Triage nurse. For some reason, this struck me as an odd term. Maybe I do not know the definition. I looked it up: "To sort out the most important cases, first used when talking about taking those from the battlefield who had a chance at survival." I waited all day. I had given her my cell phone number so I would not have to worry about missing the call. At 2:30 that afternoon, Joann called. "Dr. Sterling said, 'That's fine.'" "What's fine?" I could not believe my ears. Joann went on, "It's fine to wear the adductor at night. That's the question you asked." "No, that is not the question I asked." I am certain I was barely concealing my frustration. "Well, that's what it says here." "I am not sure why it says that, that is not what I told Carla." Enough of this, I thought. "Would it be possible to have Dr. Sterling himself call me?" "No, he's in surgery on Tuesdays." I reminded her as gently as I could, "No, actually, he's in surgery on Mondays." "Oh, you are right. I am not sure where he is, but he is gone for the day."

Before I could formulate a plea that might prevent another sleepless night, Joann offered to page Dr. Sterling and explain the situation. Thank you.

I waited. And waited. By 6:30 p.m., the doctors' office was long closed. Since I had not received a call from Dr. Sterling, I was certain he had not gotten the message. I decided to call the after hour's number. Dr. Blasire was on call. Sh**. OK, I am desperate — maybe he will act as if he cares.

He called back right away. I was two sentences into my explanation when he cut me off saying, "This is not an emergency, call back during business hours and talk to Dr. Sterling." Snap — I could almost hear it. "That is precisely what I did today." "Well, I don't know why he didn't call you back. It's his practice." I see. Actually, I did not see at all. "But it's not an emergency, and he'll have to answer those questions." He had not even let me ask *those* questions. Years of fighting with men like this who think they are God gave me the courage to say, "I am sorry that you don't view this with any urgency, but we have been without sleep for too long. I do not want to undo the results of the surgery, and I need to know if it is OK to leave off the braces and pillow to allow us all to sleep or else I need some sleep medication." He came back with an annoyed, "I usually give Valium for that." "He's already taking Valium." "The only other thing is Benadryl." Great, I thought. I just love giving medicine that has a completely different purpose that happens to have the side effect of causing the thing you want. Arrgh. Never mind. "We have Benadryl."

"Well if you don't need any medicine, I can't help you." This statement embodies the mentality of Western medical philosophy. By some miracle, I did not scream. "Could you please explain to me who is in charge of your practice?" "It's a group practice." He added impatiently, "We're each in charge of our own practices." "Yet, you share triage nurses and patient-care coordinators, and you are on call for him." Dead silence. I ventured on, "Perhaps you could try viewing this from a parent's point of view. I tried to follow your rules. I called as soon as you opened, left messages, and got a return call that indicated that the questions were miscommunicated. When things like that happen, it must affect all of you. As soon as I realized that your office must be closed, I called the after hour's number." Still silence. He finally responded defensively, "I called you as soon as I got your page." What good did that do, I wondered to myself, and just said, "Thank you for that." I let myself have a rare, completely un-Christian venting. "What an a** h***," I thought. "Go to H***, Dr. Blasire. Go directly to H*** and do not pass Go." Later, I more kindly thought, "I pray to God that you or a loved one are never on the receiving end of your kind of 'care.'"

"Never Discuss Politics or Religion"

I get in trouble a lot regarding politics. I have all but stopped talking about politics because of that. People get angry quickly if someone does not agree with them. I hesitated to put anything about politics in this book, but I think it is important to share at least a bit about how I came to believe what I believe. Perhaps if more people thought about why they believe what they believe, they would not get so angry with dissenters.

I want to start by saying that I do not know anyone who does not want every person to have food, shelter, education, health care, and meaningful work. These are basic needs for most people. I do not know anyone who disputes that. What we disagree on is *how* to ensure these needs, that is, the policies (hence the term politics) that should be in place to ensure them.

As a preface to this section involving some unpleasant letters and stories, I would like to say that while the free market is not perfect, my journey with Ryan has taught me that BY FAR the worst experiences we have ever had with medicine or law have been when a government-run agency has been involved.

Another thing most people would agree on is that Ryan is in the class of the most vulnerable of human beings. Fortunately for Ryan, Larry, Zulfi, and I have all worked hard and been able to take care of him. One of the most frustrating things for me was how often Ryan was denied services because we made "too much money." While I could understand an income limit for eligibility, I could never understand why these agencies could not figure out how to let us pay for the service, which was often not available anywhere else.

Doctors and Lawyers, Western-Style
Waiting

One of the first letters I wrote as Ryan's advocate was to speak out about the amount of time doctors expect us to wait and their hypocritical policies when patients are late.

At the time, we still lived farther out, so we were driving 30 to 45 minutes to get almost anywhere. In traffic, the doctor's office was closer to 45 minutes away. Kiran was a baby, and Ryan was seven. It had been a rough morning, and it took a great deal for me to get both kids ready and make it to the doctor on time.

As I signed in, struggling with both children, the assistant said, "The doctor is running two hours behind."

"Excuse me?" "Yes, it has been one of the 'those' days." I wanted to scream, "Tell me about it!" I said instead, "I wish someone had called me. It was very difficult to get here, and now I have to wait with two kids for two hours." The assistant was indignant; "We don't have time for that."

Unusual for me at the time, I responded quickly with, "Do you think I have time to wait for two hours? I could be doing many things that are more productive than waiting here." She just looked away. Above her head, I noticed the sign "We reserve the right to cancel your appointment if you are more than 15 minutes late." I snapped inside. I sat down with Ryan and Kiran and made the best of our long wait. And I resolved to do something about this.

I waited a while to write the letter so that it would be polite. I explained that I understand that emergencies happen, sick visits happen, etc., but if a doctor is running late, a call to the patient shows the same respect that the sign indicates that the doctor's office expects.

I got a polite letter in response back. As a result of my letter, other similar letters, and some related experiences, the office hired a new office manager and was studying how to improve its practices. Even given the nature of medical care, it is not impossible for doctors' offices to run on time. I have never waited more than 15 minutes for our neurologist, for example. Our dentist's office has called before when the doctor was running late (unusual) or early (someone had canceled) to see if we would prefer an earlier time.

Encouraged by this positive result, I began to speak out more often when things were "wrong."

Here is one of the letters:

Theresa Jeevanjee
St. Louis, MO 63129

April 25, 1999

Jorge Sergio, M.D.
St. Louis, MO 63017

Dear Dr. Sergio,

I wanted to take some time to write a letter regarding some things about your office, which I think are important.

First, I would like to say how happy we have always been with Dr. Marsha. She has been our pediatrician since my son, Ryan Maxwell, was born in 1990. She has always been a very special doctor. My son has an extremely rare chromosome disorder, which she always takes into consideration when giving him care. She always takes time to answer any questions or concerns we may have, and has often gone "above and beyond the call of duty." We know we are very fortunate to have such a wonderful pediatrician and wanted to tell you.

You have many special doctors at your practice. Besides you, we have found that Dr. Inez Hung and Dr. Papito are also exceptional pediatricians. I have always been impressed that when I call your office around 8 am (sometimes a couple minutes before you actually open), you cheerfully answer the phone, take a message, answer a question, or make an appointment as though it were the most important thing you had to do all day. I really appreciate this because this is often the most convenient time for me to call. I am sure that you are very busy at that time of day, but it never comes across in your tone of voice.

I wish I could say the same about your administrative staff. There have been many times over the last nine years that if I thought I could get the same level of care for my son that Dr. Marsha gives us, I would have left the practice.

I realize your staff must be very busy, but I don't think it takes any more time to be courteous than it does to be rude. The general attitude does not seem to be one appropriate for administrative staff working for patients and their parents, but rather irritation. I am sorry that I do not have specific names because it is likely that it does not apply to everyone. I have many examples, but a few especially frustrating ones, two very recent and one which happened over a year ago.

Over a year ago, after a very bad fall, my son started having seizures and was hospitalized. Dr. Marsha was on maternity leave at the time. Normally, because all of your doctors are good, I gladly accept whichever doctor is on call. At this time, however, I felt very strongly that Dr. Marsha should be consulted because of the fact she always remembers "little things" that are not written in the chart. She has often caught subtle problems that other doctors miss.

The person who answered the phone was very rude to me and insistent that Dr. Marsha was on maternity leave. When I asked to talk to her supervisor, I was greeted with someone who was equally as curt. She identified herself as Mrs. Sergio. I tried to explain the situation and asked simply that Dr. Marsha be consulted by whoever was covering for her. The response was, "Well, only because we have to call her about something else will we mention it." Later, Dr. McKinley told me that he was also impressed by Dr. Marsha's memory of details about Ryan. He commented, "I had Ryan's chart in my hand and *she* was 'reading' it to *me*."

Not too long ago, I waited an hour and a half to see a doctor. I certainly understand that there are valid reasons for doctors getting behind: taking extra time to answer questions and concerns, returning emergent and urgent phone calls, and seeing very sick patients who had to be "worked in." Getting behind is often unavoidable since patient care must be put before schedules.

Waiting a short time is acceptable and easy to handle. Waiting for a long time is very frustrating. In addition to having kids in the waiting room for that amount of time, there are usually many things to rearrange in order to get to the doctor. I had gotten another teacher to cover the course I teach at Saint Louis University, rushed to get my son at school, rushed home to pick up my daughter and was told that the doctor is running 45 minutes behind. When I asked why someone hadn't called to let me know, I was snapped at, "We don't have time for that."

The irritation and words both sent the message that your patients' and their parents' time is not valued or even considered. Does it really take that much time to call patients if a doctor is running significantly behind? I know your patients' parents would appreciate it. My dentist office does it if they are running more than 15 minutes behind.

This past Saturday, I called to make a sick visit for my son. Dr. Papito had seen our daughter, Kiran, the Tuesday before and given her Zithromax for an ear infection. She told us to check back before getting the refill to see whether Dr. Marsha wanted to continue it another five days. I tried to make an appointment at the same time to have her ears checked and was told "We can take a sick visit, but the ear recheck will have to wait."

We live 45 minutes from your office and making separate appointments not only meant two long trips, but more time off work. I explained this to the receptionist and was told with an irritated tone, "We only have two doctors covering for seven." I was very frustrated at hearing this. I can understand the necessity for these rules, but it takes less than five minutes to check an ear infection and it would have saved me time off work and an hour and a half round-trip drive. And, even if this had to be the final decision, it could have been delivered in a much nicer tone. I was, once again, left with the feeling that my children and my time were not valued by the administrative staff.

Again, let me say that we are extremely pleased with the care we have received from the doctors at your practice. I wanted to bring these other matters to your attention because of how important the administrative staff is to the work of the doctors. Thank you for taking the time to read this and consider my suggestions.

Sincerely,

Theresa Jeevanjee

Cc: Dr. Marsha

Things Improved Remarkably After those Letters:

Theresa Jeevanjee

St. Louis, MO 63129

August 9, 1999

Pediatric Office Manager

Dear Ms. S,

I wanted to follow up my letter dated April 25, 1999 and our subsequent phone conversation.

I have noticed an improvement in the attitudes of your staff and the general "flow" of office procedures. My recent experiences of making or changing appointments, one urgent call to the office, one call to the exchange, and bringing in our children have all been very pleasant.

Thank you for your part in this. I hope you will pass along my appreciation to those involved and to Dr. Sergio.

Sincerely,

Theresa Jeevanjee

(Mother of Ryan Maxwell, Kiran, and Lauren Jeevanjee)

Theresa Jeevanjee, Ph.D.

Webster Groves, MO 63119

February 12, 2002

Jorge Sergio, M.D.
St. Louis, MO 63017

Dear Dr. Sergio,

I just wanted to compliment your office on how efficiently it "runs." We have not had to wait for more than 15 minutes to be seen in a very long time. This is something I really appreciate, not just because we are all busy, but because when I am waiting, it is usually with three kids.

Today was an especially pleasant visit. Dr. Greer has been covering for Dr. Marsha the past several times we have been to your office. She is almost always on time, but never rushes. Today, we were early; were seen right away; and were out of the office a minute or two after our scheduled time to arrive.

It is also nice to know that my kids do not mind going to the doctor. I am sure this is due, in large part, to Drs. Marsha, Greer, and Inez. You really do have a wonderful group of doctors.

I've noticed that the staff at the front desk is friendlier, too. Thank you for whatever you have done to improve things over the years.

Sincerely,

Theresa Jeevanjee

(Mother of Ryan Maxwell, Kiran and Lauren Jeevanjee)

And then Ryan turned 18

Because one usually needs a lawyer to resolve some conflict, I am grateful to say that I have had very little contact with lawyers. But, perhaps if I had more experience with them, the journey to becoming Ryan's guardian would not have been so difficult.

Everyone at his wonderful school, Southview Special School, kept telling us it was coming. They started saying this when he was 16, held workshops on becoming a guardian, and provided handouts. There were few lawyers who worked in this area, and the ones who did were very expensive. We of course made "too much money" for the state-appointed lawyers.

To this day, the way I feel about the whole ordeal is that I would have preferred to take the thousands of dollars it cost to become Ryan's legal guardian and thrown them in the street.

I have put most of the memories out of my head, except the state lawyer be-bopping up our driveway in her BMW asking, "Has Ryan been served?" I closed my eyes recalling the sad day when the police officer beat me to the bus to serve Ryan papers about his mom trying to get custody of him. Ryan was scared. I answered the waiting lawyer, "Yes." She was happy, "Good." I was not smiling, "No, it was not good." I decided to tell her how much Ryan has always loved school and the bus, and how scared he was when a police officer greeted him unexpectedly. She changed her demeanor, "Oh, I'm sorry, I didn't realize. I just meant …" We had a better relationship after that, and she ended up teaching my (highly paid) lawyer what to do.

As for the whole experience, it left me numb. After we "won," we were ushered into an office that was too small for three people. A different state-appointed lawyer, who was in charge of the next step, was gushing about how I needed to "stop thinking like a mom, and start thinking like a guardian." I thought, "What an idiot," but said nothing. Zulfi took my hand.

As we left, Zulfi said to me, "I am surprised you didn't say something to him." I smiled, "Oh, don't you remember what he said at the beginning? I just need to file a one-page report each year about how I am still taking care of MY SON, and I never have to see these people again. He's not worth it." His immediate response was, "I am proud of you."

About six months later, the lawyer I called "Ms. BMW" telephoned and left a message indicating that she was rather irritated. She had not yet been paid by the state, and her message was that I needed to pay her. I found this comical and left the following voice message on her phone:

"You are a good lawyer, and you worked hard for Ryan, convincing the State (unnecessarily in my opinion) that his mother was a fit guardian for him. You even helped my highly paid, inexperienced lawyer get through this. You deserve to get paid. In fact, I think you deserve most of the money I paid him in addition to the amount the State should have paid you. However, I am not going to pay you both. I have already paid my lawyer over $6,000. If I can help you get paid by the State, I would be happy to do so."

She returned my call and said, "You are right. I will work harder on getting them to pay me."

Another Interesting Conversation

Yes, everything changed when Ryan turned 18. At least it seemed that way.

I answered the call, which caller ID indicated was long distance, with a simple, "Hello."

"My name is Jean Garlic (not her real name). I am Ryan Maxwell's insurance advocate. May I please speak to him?"

I started to say, "I am Ryan's mother …."

She cut me off, "Ryan is 18 now, I need to speak with him in person."

I tried again, "But he is unable to …."

"I must insist."

After a couple more unsuccessful attempts to say that Ryan is mentally and physically handicapped, and consequently does not communicate beyond the level of a toddler, I handed the phone to Ryan. Zulfi just looked at me incredulously.

"Hi!" Ryan said in his friendly, excited way, "Howareyoooooo?" When Ryan asks 'how are you,' it all runs together like one very happy word. If you ask him how he is, he usually replies, "I'm *pine*, howar-eyoooo?" Howareyoooo, again. One happy, infinite loop.

I could not hear Ms. Garlic's response, but Ryan kept repeating "Hi!" and "Howareyooooo?" Occasionally, there would be a pause, and he would ask, "Huh?" Zulfi, still in the kitchen at the time, asked, "How long are you going to let this go on?" I thought that was obvious, "Until the point is made."

After about five minutes, which I am fairly certain seemed longer to Ms. Garlic, I took the phone, and a very relieved and apologetic "advocate" said quickly, "I am sorry, can we start over?" We can always start over.

Circa 2013

To Whom It May Concern:

After a very frustrating time of trying to navigate MO Health Net's phone system and website, I was told I must download the form for appointing an authorized representative so that I could find out why MO Health Net is being asked information by UHC (please see enclosed). While I appreciate the policy involved, this form does not ensure what the policy intends, that is, to ensure that individuals do in fact give permission to their representatives.

Even after explaining that my son, Ryan Maxwell, is mentally retarded and physically disabled, and that I am his legal guardian, I was told I needed this form before anyone could talk with me. The form (also enclosed) is intended to be completed and signed by Ryan. As his legal guardian, I complete and sign forms for him since he is not able to do so. So, I completed and signed the form (as Ryan) to authorize myself to be his representative. And then I signed the form again (as myself) saying that I am willing to act on his behalf. I am sure you can see how unnecessary and ineffective this is.

I am writing to make you aware that there seems to be a "hole" in the process because I am quite sure Ryan is not the only adult you serve who cannot sign for himself and this form presents an easy opportunity for fraud. Since I had to send in certified copies of legal guardianship and other proof of disability when we applied for MO Health Net services, I am not sure why that would not have been adequate to have me be an authorized representative. I hope that a copy of proof of legal guardianship is adequate support of the inadequate form. If not, please let me know what else is necessary.

Sincerely,

Theresa L. Jeevanjee

Here We Go Again

Linda, (a friend of mine who is also a lawyer)

Found the email with the lawyer's names, thanks. I will call these guys Monday. The problem is that it is unchartered territory except for these Public attorneys, and what a nightmare that has been already.

I would appreciate it if you keep your ears and eyes open for a lawyer experienced with this. I'm going to summarize the situation because it's not really a social security disabilities problem, at least not ONLY that.

Ryan (at 23) is a legal adult. I am his legal guardian (another nightmare that was ...). He has no assets but receives social security disability, a very small amount, not enough to live on, which for now is not a worry since he has us. He receives funding through a Medicaid waiver (essentially the system through which these services are paid is called a waiver — I have asked till I'm blue in the face why it's called a waiver ...) and the DMH (Department of Mental Health). The former pays for AADD (Association on Aging with Developmental Disabilities) for part-time care, and the latter pays for Sarah Care part time. Together they add up to his allowed funding, actually a bit under. He needs both programs because AADD is too expensive, and too much activity and Sarah Care is too sedentary; he benefits from a mix. Besides, I have been told the better waiver to have is Medicaid for when we are gone. Unfortunately, we cannot drop Sarah Care because of our schedules, so we need both programs. Sarah Care has applied for three years to be funded through Medicaid waiver and has been put off — system overload.

Last year the state made an arbitrary decision that services can only be funded through one waiver and simultaneously stopped allowing agencies to apply for new waivers! Lots of folks lost services. I appreciate the state's motive to save money. However, they are disregarding situations like Ryan's (and many folks are in these split situations). The policy the State created references the Social Security Law section 1915c (don't quote that — I am going from memory), but I downloaded the entire law in PDF and searched for keywords, and the law does NOT say anything about limiting waivers.

I appealed once and got an extension. And then without notice, they canceled the waiver that funds Sarah Care, even though I have a letter saying that it will be funded until June 2014. So, here we go again. The second lawyer I called gave up and told me to call Eastern Missouri Legal Services. I have been trying to get a call back from them for two weeks. Yesterday at 6 pm they finally called only to say "we only do up until 19 years old, I'll have someone call you Monday." I really don't have a lot of faith in that.

While I don't have faith in the state's legal service system, I'm worried about the cost of another lawyer if it's not through ARAG.

I just got the bill for Sarah Care, which is $900. And while we live well, with me not working, adding $900 a month plus a good deal more for a lawyer would be tough. Anyway, I'm only mentioning this to say that we would ask a lawyer to base his/her fee on Ryan's income or mine, not Zulfi's.

Please let me know if any of this doesn't make sense and/or if you can recommend anyone. Meantime, I will call the other two lawyers you mentioned.

I hope asking your advice is not an abuse of our friendship. I just don't know what else to do. I am also very worried about what will happen when we are gone.

In deep gratitude,

Theresa

Mr. Furr, (not his real name)

Thanks for taking the time to discuss this today. Attached are the PDF docs I have. I am going to summarize the situation below in case it helps. Thanks for your consideration.

Theresa

Summary:

I am legal guardian and mother of Ryan Maxwell, who has a rare chromosome disorder that manifests itself in mental retardation and physical handicaps. Currently he spends about half of his week with AADD (Association on Aging with Developmental Disabilities) and the other half with Sarah Care. The former is funded via Medicaid Waiver and the latter is funded though a DMH Waiver. For reasons I can explain if you like, Ryan needs a mix of both of these programs. Sarah Care has tried to apply for funding though Medicaid, but they stopped taking new providers when this new State Law came into effect.

The State "law" states that clients cannot receive funding through more than one waiver and quotes the Social Security law section 1915c. I have read it several times, downloaded it and searched the file – it does not say "no two waivers" anywhere.

As you can see from the docs, I appealed the first decision and seemed to win at least an extension. By the way it was a very frustrating experience. The letter I first got said that funding would continue if I appealed, which I did, and then I got a call saying, "We don't care, we are cutting off funding anyway." It took me three days to get a person on the phone to agree that this was not right and to extend funding as the letter agreed. And then in January, 2014, after the appeal extending until June, they cut funding off again without notice by leaving a message on our phone.

We have never received funding for Ryan until we were forced to when he turned 18. We have worked hard and have enjoyed an above average middle income life style. If we did not pay so much in taxes, we could afford to pay for this care of Ryan. Care of people with disabilities is awful in this state (country, world), and I think both political parties share in the blame. If we were not taxed so much, we could afford for his care. And this relatively high income that puts us in a high tax bracket denies us eligibility for services he needs. Penalized either way.

I hope this makes sense. Please let me know if I can clarify anything. And thanks in advance for your time in reviewing this.

Thank you very much for your time.

Theresa

We received a letter that Mr. Furr could not help us because he assists clients to prove that they are disabled. I was saddened and discouraged that yet another lawyer I had hoped could help us could not, but I was even more saddened and discouraged that a highly paid lawyer is necessary to PROVE that people are disabled.

Our Tax Dollars at Work

I include this petition as an example of the sort of thing that is sometimes necessary to advocate for a person with a disability. In case the reader cannot follow it, I sympathize. I have gone through it several times, and it is hard for me to follow. I am not trying to solicit sympathy, rather to bring awareness.

1.   Petitioner is a resident of St. Louis County, Missouri. He brings this action by his mother and guardian, Dr. Theresa Jeevanjee. Petitioner is 24 years old and has been diagnosed with the chromosomal defect Partial Trisomy 12 and mental retardation. Petitioner is incontinent, engages in only limited speech and is unable to care for himself independently.

2.   Petitioner was previously determined by the Department of Social Services, Family Support Division to be eligible for services under the Missouri Medicaid ("MO HealthNet") program. Through his participation in the MO HealthNet program, Petitioner was deemed eligible to receive Adult Day Care ("ADC") services, which are administered by the Department of Health and Senior Services ("DHSS"), Division of Senior and Disability Services ("DSDS").

3.   As an individual with a developmental disability, Petitioner was also determined eligible for certain types of medical assistance through the MO HealthNet Home and Community-Based Services ("HCBS") Community Support Waiver program, which is administered by the Department of Mental Health ("DMH"), Division of Developmental Disabilities ("DD").

4.   On May 29, 2013, Respondent issued Petitioner an Adverse Notice for Home and Community Based Services ("Adverse Notice"), which stated Petitioner's ADC services would be discontinued "due to… [§]1915(c) of the Social Security Act: [i]ndividuals may only be enrolled

in one Home and Community Based Waiver at a time, regardless of which state agency." exhibit __.

5.   Petitioner timely requested an administrative hearing to review Respondent's determination on June 4, 2013. exhibit___.

6.   A hearing was conducted on July 22, 2013 in front the Missouri Department of Social Services ("DOSS"), MO HealthNet Division ("Division"). Respondent was represented by Sandra Stith of the Missouri Department of Health and Senior Services ("DHSS"), Division of Senior and Disability Services ("DSDS"). exhibit___.

7.   During the hearing, Respondent claimed the determination to terminate services was based on an excerpt from the Home and Community Based Services Manual, Appendix 1, Legal References for Adverse Action, which states that §1915(c) of the Social Security Act indicates that individuals may only be enrolled in one HCBS at a time, regardless of which state agency is administering that waiver. exhibit __.

8.   Respondent never entered the text of §1915(c) of the Social Security Act into the administrative record.

9.   Respondent never requested the hearing officer to take judicial notice of the existence or contents of §1915(c) of the Social Security Act or any other statutes, regulations, rules, or policies.

10.   Petitioner never stipulated to the existence, terms or applicability of the law or any other statutes, regulations, rules, or policies.

11.   In fact, Petitioner, through his guardian Dr. Jeevanjee, presented testimony that she was unable to locate any language prohibiting an individual's participation in more than one waiver in either §1915(c) or the entirety of §1915 of the Social Security Act, even after conducting a "PDF" word search for the language quoted by Respondent within the document. exhibit __. (p.12)

12.   Petitioner's father Larry Maxwell also presented testimony that despite reading all of §1915 from "cover to cover," he was also unable to

locate any language in the cited law that would support Respondent's position that an individual "may only be enrolled in one HCBS waiver at a time". exhibit ___. (p.12)

13.   During the hearing, Respondent's representative Sandra Stith was repeatedly asked to identify where in §1915 the language cited by Respondent in the Home and Community Based Services Manual, Appendix 1, Legal References for Adverse Action was located. In the alternative, Ms. Stith was asked to identify any other sources of authority such as agency policies, rules or regulations that would support Respondent's assertion that an individual could not be enrolled in more than one HCBS waiver. exhibit ___. (p.12, 15, 16)

14.   Ms. Stith testified, " I'm not the official person from my bureau of programs integrity which is our Policy Unit...and they develop our polices based on laws and regulations that we have to follow of the services that we do provide to our participants...I'll have to forward that information to our Bureau of Program Integrity, our Policy Unit, for a more specific answer in reference to how – where it is found in the law – that I believe your question is where it's found in the law on the Adverse Action Notice...as far as stating that person cannot be authorized for two waivers." exhibit ___. (p. 15)

15.   In response to Petitioner's questioning of Ms. Stith, the hearing officer also offered certain testimony sua sponte stating, "I obviously will look at where that is in the Social Security Act since you're raising that... the other thing that will often come into play is that there are also regulations, so a lot of the time, the Act will essentially just say, you know, this is what the policy is...and then you have to go down a few levels into the regulations." exhibit ___. (p. 12)

16.   Division rendered a decision upholding the termination of Petitioner's ADC benefits on December 30, 2013.

17.   Petitioner timely appealed Division's decision on January 16, 2014.

Status

As of this writing, we have spent over a year, and many thousands of dollars, disputing what is an illegal policy decision by the State.

We are waiting. It makes me very worried not only for Ryan's future, but also especially for the future of those with disabilities who have no one to advocate for them.

6

Advocating for Myself

*"Put your own oxygen mask on first,
then assist those around you."*
– General airplane wisdom.

Put on Your Own Oxygen Mask First

That advice seems so simple and logical. How could you possibly help someone else if you cannot breathe yourself? Yet we so often deplete ourselves of everything, including oxygen, while giving to those we love, especially our children. Most parents I know have no trouble taking care of their children. Many are even taking care of other people's children and their own aging parents, as well.

It took me a long time, and several years of counseling, to take care of myself and many more to be an advocate for myself. My counselor taught me to stop saying selfish and instead to think of things I do for myself as *self-FULL*. Like breathing, I am filling myself so that I can help others, and even when I'm not helping others, to be my full self.

Being Alone (All One) is Essential

I love to be alone; it is the best way for me to regenerate. It is why I run — usually alone. Running is not just physical for me; it's spiritual. Time to pray, think, energize. It's also why I try to go on a retreat by myself once a year. I am not sure how I found Mt. St. Francis friary in Indiana, but I have been there several times. Sometimes I even wrote about it.

November 7, 2003

My Dearest Ryan,

This letter probably does not belong here – I may delete it, but for now it seems a fitting place for a personal note from me as I was trying to add more to your book.

I am at Mt. St. Francis in Indiana. It is a conventional Franciscan Friary and Retreat House. It has been lovely to just be alone.

I have eaten, slept, gone to every prayer service and mass.

I have graded papers, taken walks and stared out the window. No one has tugged on me, I have not had to referee fights, and I have not had to ask for anything. This must be what heaven is like (modulo the grading papers part).

Coming here has given me a very necessary chance to reset after last Wednesday night, which was awful. In the span of two hours I was told that my father was dying and that, despite all of our efforts, you would likely need hamstring surgery after all.

Two separate issues, each needing more emotional and physical energy than I had at the time since I was going on over three weeks of too little sleep. I know that I will be given the strength to deal with the issues as well as the necessary support. I have so many wonderful people in my life, and I know that God will provide. But sometimes I just want to scream, "Enough!" Just for today, I would like to bask in the sunshine and know that I have learned enough, that I am strong enough, and that I have given enough. I suppose that sounds arrogant, and, deep down, I do know that as long as there are lessons being offered, I must need them.

You have been my greatest teacher, my greatest love, my toughest challenge. Thank you with all of my heart and soul for allowing me the privilege and honor of being your mom.

A counselor I saw for many years during some very rough years shared that she believed our children choose their parents. I do not know, but it is a very nice thought that out of all the moms you could have had, you chose me. I know that I am not perfect, but I hope that you know how much I love you and that I have always tried to be a good mom.

I am not ready to let you go; I never will be, but I think when I am older and wiser, it might be a little easier. I still need you.

Please do not die if you need to have surgery. Please do not stop walking! We have worked too hard for you to crawl and walk to give it up. I know that you do not want to give up walking – that is why you were so sad until we found Sue. Please hang in there with us – it will get better.

Yours forever,

Mommy

November 16, 2007

Dearest Ryan,

Here I am once again at Mt. St. Francis Retreat Center. I came another time in between this and 2003, but I don't think I worked on your book then. I have as one of my sabbatical goals to add 2,000 words. We will see. When I think of all the wonderful authors, I wonder whether I will even get anyone to consider publishing it.

So much has happened that I hardly know where to begin. I suppose I should start with the major surgery you had in July and then go backwards. It still seems so fresh. Thinking about it gives me "writer's block." I think I will revisit this later.

November 16, 2007 (later)

My dear son, you will turn 18 in April. That seems unfathomable. On your 16th birthday, we had a "see what love can do" party. We called it that because I was sharing with someone that doctors predicted that if you made it through the week (which was unlikely), you would not live past age 4. Her response was, "see what love can do." Since 16 is the square of 4, it seemed a great time to say, "hah, take that, see what love can do!" We had a grand party with carriage rides. You got on the carriage, and I pulled you off 3.5 hours later to change you and give you a sandwich. You rode the last half hour, too. Anyone who wanted to see you had to ride the carriage.

Our friend, Amy, made a video of your life from pictures. We had one looping on the t.v. and one on a mini t.v. outside. There was not a dry eye in the place. I still cannot watch it without crying.

I knew the party was a success when you woke up the next day and asked, "bird day pardy?" You wanted another one. God willing, we will have another on 21 and 30 and 40 and .... Maybe we will do a smaller version with just carriage rides for 18.

You love to ride around in all kinds of vehicles. You also like to ride horses. Perhaps it is because I ran during your (and the girls') pregnancy and you like being jostled. You remind us all to take joy in simple pleasures. Being here at the "The Mount" does remind me to take time out and live more simply. I smile as I type this on my laptop ... Still it is much more simple than the fast-paced life we lead.

I have been on sabbatical this semester. Sabbatical comes from the word Sabbath – a rest in your seventh year. It has been truly restorative and restful. I have worked, worked hard, but nothing compared to the usual chaos that is the academic life. And I have completed a good number of non-work related projects as well. It is so nice to have time for painting and writing and just being.

Love,
Mom

Dancing

There is a picture of me in a pink tutu smiling. I am tall enough to be six, but Mom says I was only three or four in the picture. In my mind, I have always loved ballet. Mom told me that when I was three, she took me to a ballet class, and I cried. She never took me back. If she were alive, I might protest, "But I was only three! Who listens to three-year-olds?!" If I let Kiran stop ballet every time she wanted to in the first two years, she would not be the beautiful dancer she is today. She and I are so glad I made her stick with it. I told her, "You need to give it three years, after that if you still want to quit, you may." She never did.

After many years of sitting in the lobby or hallway waiting for Kiran and/or Lauren to finish ballet class, I decided to take a class myself. One does not begin ballet in one's 40s and hope to achieve anything lofty, but I stuck with it. It has been very therapeutic.

I wrote the following in 2014 after many lessons and dances with Ryan.

There is a poem, "Everything important in life, I learned in kinder-garten." When I read that, I thought, "That's what's wrong with me — I never went to kindergarten." It was optional in those days, and since my older brother went and was bored in first grade, my mother decided I should skip it.

I started taking ballet (something else I did not get to do when young) regularly in my forties. I would submit, that "Everything important in life, I learned in ballet."

- Ballet is beautiful; so is Life.
- It takes sacrifice, discipline, and practice.
- To be able to dance for just 15 to 30 minutes, it takes 45 minutes to an hour of warm up and preparation.
- Anything worthwhile takes a lot of preparation and practice.
- You end class by "reverence," a slow, graceful dancing "bow" to say thank you to the teacher and the pianist (if you are lucky enough to have one).
- Even when it hurts, you have to keep going.
- Self-esteem is the reward for hard work and discipline; it is earned, not given.

- But it's not enough to just keep going. You must also smile like it is easy.
- It is rarely easy.

The people who do ballet are among the most disciplined, hard working and beautiful people I know, inside and out. Ballet bodies are the best; they reflect the hard work and appreciation for beauty that it takes to do ballet. Our bodies almost always reflect what we do in life. The show must go on. It simply must.

This weekend when I went to check on three of my daughters, two biological and one of my several "adopted" ones, they were all sprawled out on the beds, tummies showing and in the flexible positions that only ballerinas could sleep in. I thought, "They are so beautiful." Their bodies reflect the hard work they have done all these years. As I was enjoying the pretty sight, I reflected how grateful I am that we could provide all the training and lessons that ballet gives. Life is Beautiful, So Is Ballet.

More on Dancing

I believe this so strongly, which is why my email signature includes one of these quotes:

"I get up. I walk. I fall down. Meanwhile, I keep dancing."

– Daniel Hillel

"Hard times require furious dancing."

– Alice Walker

Dancing has been one of the ways that I have taken care of myself. Dance class remains one of the best (and relatively inexpensive) forms of therapy I know.

Late at night (or early in the morning), I will often "dance with my mop" as I clean the kitchen floor. Once, my niece, Brooke, who was visiting for Christmas, caught me in the kitchen and went and told her father (my brother Kenny). "Auntie Teri is dancing with the mop, Daddy." "That's OK, that's how Aunt Teri copes."

Running

Long before I took my first dance class, I was a runner. Some will tell you that dancers cannot or should not run. And anyone who sees me dance will probably tell you runners cannot dance (at least this one). Oh well. I do a great many things I "should" not or should not be able to do. I used to run as a teen with my older brother, George. And then in college, I became a "serious" runner after taking a course in aerobics (back when physical education was still required in college). We had to read Kenneth Cooper's new (at the time) book, and I was hooked on running from then on.

I will go without many things in order to run. I will, and often do, rearrange my entire day to fit in running. Sometimes this means doing an inside run around my house — it's silly but better than the treadmill.

Running is not just good for me physically; it is spiritual AllOne time and time in nature (unless I'm running inside, of course.) It also keeps my (undiagnosed) ADHD in check. Well, mostly.

For some reason in my life, there have been many questions or tests that ask me to choose one word to define myself. If I am honest, the one word has to be mathematician (I am logical to a fault) followed closely by artist and runner. Mathematicians are not usually artists (equal mix of left and right brain is not common). Sometimes it would be nice not to be so unusual. If someone asked me what word I would *like* to identify myself, it would be dancer, followed closely by poet.

Taking time to be AllOne, taking time to be with family and friends (especially if I can mix these with eating good food), running, dancing, painting, and praying. These are my oxygen masks.

7

Angels Among Us

For he commands his angels with regard to you,
to guard you wherever you go.
– Psalms 91:11
http://www.usccb.org/bible

and

You are Special

...The LORD called me, from my mother's womb he gave me my name.
He made my mouth like a sharp-edged sword ....He said to me, You are
my servant, ... For now the LORD has spoken, who formed me as his
servant from the womb, ...
– Isaiah 49:1-5
http://www.usccb.org/bible

Angels Among Us

I love the movie *Fried Green Tomatoes*. It is such a good story for many reasons. It portrays friendship, loyalty, love, community, and justice in ways that few stories do. As I have mentioned before, my favorite quote from that movie is "It's a well-known fact that there are angels on earth masqueradin' as humans." The rest of that quote is, "And yo' momma is one of them." I am not an angel, but I am *very real* thanks to my journey with Ryan. My journey with him has convinced me that not only is he a miracle; He is also an angel masquerading as a human. A very cute human, I might add.

Real

Real in life is similar to the term normal in mathematics. It has many meanings and can mean everything from authentic to cool.

I have a copy of the following excerpt from *The Velveteen Rabbit* framed and sitting on my desk. The copy itself is "real," having been typed on a typewriter on plain paper (to give you some idea of how old it is) and faded from the sun. It reminds me that suffering is important.

I thank Ryan, from the bottom of my heart for letting me be his mom and for helping me to become *Real*.

From *The Velveteen Rabbit* by Margery Williams:

"Real isn't how you are made," said the Skin Horse. "It's a thing that happens to you. When a child loves you for a long, long time, not just to play with, but REALLY loves you, then you become Real."

"Does it hurt?" asked the Rabbit.

"Sometimes," said the Skin Horse, for he was always truthful. "When you are Real you don't mind being hurt."

"Does it happen all at once, like being wound up," he asked, "Or bit by bit?"

"It doesn't happen all at once," said the Skin Horse. "You become. It takes a long time. That's why it doesn't often happen to people who break easily or have sharp edges, or who have to be carefully kept. Generally, by the time you are Real, most of your hair has been loved off, and your eyes drop out and you get loose in the joints and very shabby. But these things don't matter at all, because once you are Real you can't be ugly, except to people who don't understand."

Your Baby Sister, Lauren, is a Real Angel Among Us
November, 2007

More on Lauren's Wisdom of God ...

My father is dying. This is not necessarily a sad thing, although I have not worked that out yet. Given the week I have had, I will work it out on the plane ride there.

I have never been close to him, and his lifelong bodily abuse (mostly smoking and drinking) are having their natural consequences.

On this the night, before I leave to visit him for the last time, I was talking to my girls about my impending absence. Kiran, our seven-year-old, who has met her grandfather, is sad. Lauren, our oldest soul, who is only four chronologically, has no memory of him.

She was asking questions about being alive and "not alive" in the manner of a typical four-year-old.

"Are you still alive when you die?" "No. It's different. If you are good, you go to heaven." "Well, aren't you alive in Heaven?" I am way too tired for this, I thought, but managed, "Not in the same way; it's like you are an angel."

There was a long pause while she pondered these thoughts. She concluded, "Right. When you are an angel, you are better than humans."

Then she wondered aloud, "Am I going to die?" I quietly said something she already knew, "All people eventually die, usually when they are old."

"But God will never die."

"That's right."

"Because God is always New."

I just smiled and hugged her and thanked the God who Sent her. I understood then why she and Ryan were so close.

Angel of God

For years, I have said this prayer with Ryan, leaving off the last word of the phrase for him to complete. He has always completed the sentences with the right word, the ones in brackets. Then there was the night he surprised me.

Angel of <God>

My guardian <dear>

To Whom God's <love>

Commits me <here>

Ever this <night>

Be at my <side>

To light and to guard,

To rule and to guide. <Amen>

That night, instead of "dear" when I said "My guardian ..." Ryan said, "Mommy" in that tone that he reserves just for me when he is being sweet. I hugged him a little more tightly and asked, "Is Mommy your guardian angel?" "Yeah," he said as though I obviously needed reminding.

Ryan is an angel of God. I am grateful that I am his mom.

Sleep. Or Rather the Lack of It.
Subtitle: It is my heaven anyway

It is a gift from God that I can get by with little sleep because I rarely get enough. I never have any trouble falling asleep, but once awakened, I often have trouble going back to sleep. Even when I fall back to sleep, being awakened several times during the night does not make for restful sleep.

Interestingly enough, the first two years of graduate school, Ryan and I both slept well. He went to bed about 9:00 p.m. and slept until 7:00 a.m. I went to bed about midnight and slept until he awoke. After graduation, everything changed. There was always something: marriage, the birth of Kiran and Lauren, Ryan's fall, seizures, perimenopause, seizures, menopause, seizures, stress at work, seizures, and storms of all kinds (including weather-related).

There were days, many of them, when I honestly do not know how I made it through the day. Times when I was so exhausted, I felt like I really was hovering over, rather than inside, a dead body that was moving against its will. By the grace of God and many small miracles, I walked through life sleep-deprived for many years. I managed (I hope) to give Ryan and his sisters a happy childhood and weather the storms that came with all of his medical issues. I even managed to finish my Ph.D. and spend 12 years teaching full time, including four as department chair, and achieving full professor. But I was very tired almost all of the time.

My sweet aunt, Gigi, and I are very close; I do not think we have ever shared a cross word. It is not that I think I cannot be close to those I am occasionally cross with. In fact, I think relationships can be even closer after a conflict is resolved. Gigi and I usually agree, however, on everything from our shared faith to politics and so have had few conflicts to resolve.

As I almost never did in those days, I was lamenting aloud that I was tired. "If I make it to heaven, I am going to sleep for the first thousand years." Gigi looked sympathetically at me but reminded me firmly, "*When* you get to heaven, you won't need to sleep." My response was the verbal equivalent of pouncing, "It's my heaven, and I am going to sleep. I have earned the right to sleep, and no one is going to deprive me of it. If God loves me, God will let me sleep for a thousand years." She opened her mouth as if to speak, but decided against it.

"It's Not About You"
April 12, 2014

Dear Ryan,

I have been writing you letters and stories since the first one in January 1990. There have often been long periods of time in between, sometimes years. But in 2013 I felt called to do what many have suggested, that is, to compile them, add more, and write this book. It helped that I was no longer working full time. I have been encouraged by many people who love you, some of whom have read early drafts.

But today something happened that made me realize I am not writing this book for me, at least not only for me. And it is not about me, either, at least not much. Buddy and your sisters are out of town. Our OT caregiver, Katelyn, graciously came at 6:40 am to lie with you until you got up and to take you to Sarah Care so I could go to my 7 am ACTS preparation meeting.

All through the meeting, I was tired. Heck, I am always tired. But lately, I am tired not from stress, but from writing. I had shared with the director of the ACTS retreat that I wanted to finish my book before I gave a talk. That reasoning did not make sense to her I am sure. I do not think it even makes sense to me, at least not any sense I could articulate.

The last two weeks I have felt "full" of the book. I could not stop writing. I would arrange my whole day to maximize writing time. Where was this coming from? OK, stupid question for someone who says she channels the Holy Spirit, but it felt different. I was driven like I have not felt since I was writing my dissertation.

As we were walking out of the ACTS team preparation meeting, the sweetheart Amy (another team member), and I were talking about what our prayer needs were. ([Each week we are grouped in triples to pray for each other.] Amy shared some family needs. I asked, "Please pray for safe travel for my family." She quickly added, "And your book. My other prayer group and I have been praying for your book." Aha. Then she proceeded to tell me why she thought this book was needed. I was humbled. When will I stop being surprised by the direct and powerful actions of the Holy Spirit? When will I stop being surprised by the miracles that happen as a result of prayer.

Another of the ACTS sisters responded when she heard my sharing of Amy's comment, "It's not about you." Good reminder.

You are Special

Dear Ryan,

There is a song that is played on every episode of one of your favorite kids shows, Barney. It talks about being special and being the only one. As I have mentioned elsewhere (in jest), if there is a purgatory, I think we just might get a free pass because of decades of watching the same shows over and over. Even you must be tired of them, because you are branching out to other shows.

Ryan, you are special, as are all people, and you are the only one, as I suppose is also true of all people, even identical twins. Yet, I am so tired of hearing "special" and "only one," and it has nothing to do with this lovely jingle or Barney the purple dinosaur.

You're the Only One

I wish I had a nickel for every time someone has said to me "You're the only one who has ever …" insert "thought this," "believed such," or "done that." I assure you, most of the time it is quite clear that they are not being complimentary. They are not putting me in the same class as the wonderful, brilliant pioneering leaders who were the only ones who thought, believed or did a certain thing such as Jesus, Isaac Newton, Joan of Arc, Harriet Tubman, Corrie ten Boom, Sojourner Truth, Mother Teresa, etc.

After several months of trying to find a lawyer who would help me appeal the illogical rule that caused two-thirds of Ryan's funding to be dropped without notice, I was hopeful that the last of the names my friend Linda, who is a lawyer, gave me would be one, seemingly the only one, who did this kind of law. During the phone call, he said, "In my 40 years of practice, you are the only one ..." I am not sure I even heard the rest of the sentence since I had been conditioned to believe those words preceded an insult born of not knowing how to deal with me. But wait, I caught a word or two that seemed to indicate that he meant it as a *compliment*.

We made an appointment to meet at 2:30 p.m. the following Friday, which was the same day as Ryan's dental work under anesthesia, but it was the only time for the foreseeable future. I hoped it would go well, knowing I would be pretty wiped out by then given my experience with early dentist appointments that involved anesthesia.

During that meeting, he said, "You are the only one ..." another time or two, and again he was being complimentary. Apparently, I am "quite resourceful." I am grateful God has helped me overcome my shyness and (some of) my insecurities so that I can be a strong advocate for Ryan.

We talked about all the aspects regarding the huge undertaking of suing the State of Missouri, a path I detested. We agreed that there did not appear to be any other alternatives. We talked about the chances of winning. We discussed cases that were related, even if only tangentially. We talked about the cost. In response to my concern about money, he said, "You should do this. You're very smart and resourceful. I think you could do it." I thanked him for what I thought must be high praise from him, but shared that I was told I would never win the appeal without a lawyer. He sighed, "That is probably true." During our meeting, he asked about Ryan. "I have been doing this for 40 years, and I have seen at least one of every kind of disability." "You haven't seen one like Ryan because he's the only one. Ryan is the only one in the medical literature with this particular manifestation of partial trisomy 12, and there are only eleven or so of those." I went on to explain the DNA specifics after he assured me he knew enough about genetics to understand it.

Then we had a pleasant conversation about Ryan and his sisters. He commented, "I have found that the siblings of disabled children are the neatest people." I agreed. After finding out that Kiran wanted to be a lawyer, he said, "Tell her not to." We laughed, "I have tried. We have lawyer friends who have also tried." Then after I shared a few stories where Kiran always gets what she sets her mind on, he invited her to help on the case. "It will save you money and be good experience for her."

We talked for over an hour, for which he did not charge me. Well, I thought, "Tom Kennedy, you are also in the 'you're the only one' set, and I am extremely grateful."

A Very Special New Year's Eve

I wrote a story about Lauren 14 years ago when a very tired Mom and her one-year-old (Lauren) wandered into a nearby restaurant, Cravings, in need of some good food and pampering. It looked like a nice place with good food. It occurred to me while looking at the menu that we would probably have to leave since there was nothing Lauren would likely eat. Unbeknownst to either of us at the time, the owner, Timothy Brennan, waited on us (his server had quit unexpectedly). He graciously said, "No worries, I can make her a grilled cheesed sandwich." Happy sigh from me.

There is a story about her happily devouring her grilled cheese "sammich" and many stories through the years about how she claimed that Tim is "God's chef" and "magic." And now that she is older, she has even taken lessons from him (her birthday present of choice this year). She is, perhaps, his biggest fan, and I'm a close second.

These many years later, now that Tim and I are friends, I knew when we brought Ryan with us to dinner that Tim would make Ryan whatever he wanted to eat. But I also know that Ryan (like his mom) enjoys good food and was hopeful that he would choose one of the yummy menu choices for New Year's Eve. As I read the choices, Buddy and I both expected him to say "chicken." But Ryan said, " 'teak" for steak. Happily, it came with Ryan's favorite vegetable (zucchini) and mashed potatoes, another favorite. Since Tim offered, we did allow Ryan to alter the dessert choice to his favorite — Tim's carrot cake.

As I sat there happily sipping champagne and enjoying my own delicious food, I enjoyed even more helping and watching as Ryan ate half of our appetizers, most of the bread, all of his salad, all of his "teak," vegetables, potatoes, and half the cake. What was so sweet was that after almost every bite, he stopped and said, "MMMMMM, dat's GOOOOOOOD." I wish Tim could have heard it.

Few things are more enjoyable (to me) than being with people I love, enjoying food crafted with love, and being waited on by caring and friendly folks (Ron and Tim) in a lovely atmosphere. And hearing Ryan enjoy every single bite, well, it was very, very special.

Thank you, Timothy Brennan and my dear Ryan, for making the world a better place.

Life is Good.

Facebook
November, 2014
My dearest Ryan,

I was a hard sell to Facebook, a hacker at heart and my first undergraduate degree being math and computer science before there was such a thing as computer science at most universities. I soon came to appreciate the sharing of inspirational quotes and pictures on Facebook. It was worth the occasional loss of a "friend" when I posted a strong opinion, especially about politics or religion.

The following captures a very important viewpoint about "special kids." In the same vein, I once said that what makes the Special School District special is not the kids (or at least not just them), but rather the special teachers and administrators who care for them and their education.

While I appreciate the sentiment of "it takes a special person to care for a child with special needs," I believe strongly that if I am Special at all, God and Ryan made me that way.

Thank you for letting me be your Mom. (I can hear you saying "Welcome.") Thank you for saving me.

In deep gratitude,

Mommmmmmeeeee

"It takes a special kind of person to care for a child with special needs."

A child with special needs will inspire you to be a special kind of person.

GLOBAL HYDRANENCEPHALY FOUNDATION

I sign off, dancing. I wrote this about a year ago:

There are times when one stays up beyond sleepiness, in spite of exhaustion. Listening to music, dancing. Embracing the silence, the need for solitude and singing and dancing.

Too-ra-loo-ra-loo-ra, too-ra-loo-ra-lie, too-ra-loo-ra-loo-ra

Hush, now, don't you cry,

Too-ra-loo-ra-loo-ra, too-ra-loo-ra-lie, too-ra-loo-ra-loo-ra

That's an Irish Lullaby.

Thank you for this song, Kenny Loggins.

Thank you, God, for makin' me Irish.

Life is so very Good.

Thank you, God, for making me "Ryan's Mom."

It Takes A Village, Revisited

It truly does take a village, to raise a child and to write a book. I am grateful to so many people and fear I have not named even half of the wonderful people who have made our journey better, even if only by teaching us lessons.

As I "sign off," it seems appropriate to talk about Ryan's signature stamp. I am blessed to have so many good friends. One of them, the very lovely, red-headed Irish Patty Kinealy, was over for dinner one night. She has a special relationship with all of us, but most especially with Ryan and "Pretzel," as our youngest, Lauren, is now known.

My nephew, Thiran, and his best friend, Jonah, came to visit one summer. We had a lovely time, and one especially fun night, the kids were all playing "St. Louis–opoly," the version of Monopoly adapted for St. Louis. The pretzel was invented in St. Louis, so a pretzel is one of the game pieces, the one Lauren was using. It is the only game piece that is flat, so it was hard to see. Several times throughout the night, we would hear, "Pretzel, pretzel, where is pretzel?" From then on, the name stuck. Lauren is Pretzel.

So, when Patty directed Ryan's hand to sign "love Ryan," and the heart came out as the start of a pretzel or the start of a Celtic knot (for the Irish in us), it seemed perfect, like so many events on our journey. Unbeknownst to me, Patty had shirts made for us with this symbol, and another good friend, Laura Rossmann, made the stamp. Such are the friends and family God has given me.

Grateful, grateful to be Ryan's mom in the company of all these angels. Life is Good.

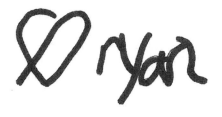

Afterword

How can we see that far?

Brad (not his real name) calls Ryan every night. Ryan knew Brad at Special School. Like Ryan, I think Brad was a bit sad and lost after graduating from Southview Special School. Calling Ryan helps them both stay connected to "bus days."

Brad's mother Sally (not her real name) is always in the background helping Brad to be polite, etc., as am I with Ryan. It is pure joy listening to their conversation. I feel like we have all become friends. I love it that Brad won't hang up without talking with "Ms. Theresa." His very sweet, "Good night, Bye-Bye" always brightens the darkest day.

Last night Sally said Brad will be going to a group home. I gasped. I did so *silently* because I would not and cannot judge, and I did not want to sound critical. It's just something that hovers in the recesses of my own mind.

Some day? We suffer from back strain and exhaustion. It's not *if*, it's *when*. Somewhere deep inside I know this, and it haunts me. As I sat in church today, holding Ryan's hand, I thought, "No one will ever love Ryan the way we do. No one will ever care for Ryan the way we do." All the time I spent wondering when and whether Ryan would die young, now I worry what happens if I go first. What if he *doesn't* die young? The thought of him in even more pain than he experiences now is the worst. I cannot see that far.

These are issues we will face all too soon. Every time I hear the ad for a nearby residence home for disabled adults on the radio that starts with "If you are the parent of an adult child with disabilities, no one has to tell you ..." No kidding. Our beloved PT, Susan, says, "That place is not safe for Ryan." I wonder if any place would be.

Meanwhile, we are still waiting to hear the outcome of our lawsuit against the State for penalizing those with disabilities. Our story is far from over. Yet, while others will say our life with Ryan is hard ... it's not hard in the way you might think. Many of our hardships are the same, or at least similar, to those that all parents have. The worry is hard. The waiting is hard. The not knowing is hard. But having Ryan in our lives? When he smiles, hugs and says things like, "Thangoo," he reminds me of how very easy it is to love him and to be part of his unusual, amazing and loving presence. We are blessed.

January, 2015

Dear Ryan,

What is next for you, then? I wonder if any place would be safe for you. No one could possibly love you like I do. Like we do. I wonder if anyone could even take adequate care of you. I worry that you will be unhappy. If we are still alive, I worry that you will feel abandoned.

Your happiness has made me and so many others happy. Losing that would make the sun stop shining, I think.

Perhaps there will be more stories with happy endings about your journey in the next book. I certainly hope so.

I love you with my whole heart,

Mommy

Glossary

Disclaimer – these terms are either words I have made up and wish to explain to the reader, explanations of acronyms that would be helpful or DNA or medical terms that I have learned through the years. While I have read a great deal and had at least two geneticists explain things to me, this is my understanding and should not be used to teach a course or explain anything where a textbook definition would be better. Any mistakes are mine.

ACTS – Adoration, Community, Theology, and Service. A renewal retreat and movement in the Catholic Church for parishes.

AllOne – the way I spell alone. Being alone is restorative for me and allows me to be One with All, especially God.

Barre – most terms in ballet are in French. Barre is the French spelling of bar, which in ballet is an actual bar attached at arms length against the wall. This is where a sequence of warm-up exercises and combinations is done every class.

Belong – in addition to spelling AllOne differently to indicate a slightly different meaning, I often capitalize words to either emphasize their meaning or to indicate that they are something more. I have never felt that I truly belong or fit in. There are many reasons for this, chief among them being I am a mathematician and an artist. A rare combination of left- and right-brain. So Belonging has been something I have longed for, but not just to fit in, to be one in being. When I think of the word, I think of wading into water and becoming the water.

Centromere – the place where chromosomes attach to form the double helix. The part above the centromere is called the "short arm," designated p, and the part below is called the "long arm," designated q.

Chromosome – In humans, there are 23 pairs of chromosomes, which can be thought of as groups of genes. We can think of the DNA strand (genome) as a book, each chromosome as a chapter, and each gene as a word or letter. It is mind boggling to consider the thousands of genes organized into chromosomes in a single intertwined double helix in EACH cell of our bodies.

Chromosomes are numbered in reverse order of size (more or less); number 1 being relatively large and 23 being much smaller. The larger the chromosome, the greater the abnormality. The normal number for each chromosome is two, each parent contributing one of the pair. So, in the case of missing chromosomal material, the term is **monosomy** (for one), and in the case of extra, the term is **trisomy** (for three).

DNA – **d**eoxyribo**n**ucleic **a**cid, is a molecule that encodes and informs development and functioning in all living organisms. In humans, this has the structure of 23 pairs of chromosomes, one from each parent, twisted in a double helix.

Modulo – an arithmetic operation that gives the remainder after dividing (or subtracting) something. The example in the book was "This must be what heaven is like (modulo grading papers)."

Monosomy – chromosomes naturally occur in pairs, one from each parent. If part of or a whole chromosome is missing, the condition is known as mono (one) somy (short for chromosome). Monosomy conditions are rarely viable since so many genes are missing. **Trisomy** – this is the condition when there is an extra part or whole chromosome.

Partial Trisomy 12 – Ryan's unique chromosome abnormality. There are only a dozen or so in the medical literature, and they are all different, that is, the extra chromosome material is either a different part of chromosome 12 or it is attached to a different chromosome.

Ryan's abnormality came about because his biological father Larry, has a **balanced translocation** between chromosomes 8 and 12.

A **balanced translocation** means that during conception, the chromosomes break apart and come together out of place. In Larry, part of chromosome 12 attached itself to chromosome 8. This can happen when eggs are old, that is, when a woman has her first child later in life. For some reason, it happens less often for subsequent children later in life.

While the condition is balanced in Larry, Ryan got a complete 12 and the chromosome 8 with the extra 12 on it. Even though it is only part, chromosome 12 is relatively large, so it is a great many genes. This has resulted in what medical science calls **MMR, moderate mental retardation**, and physical handicaps. Please see also April 27, 1990 letter for a description of when I first learned about this condition in Ryan.

Pyloric stenosis – The pylorus is a muscular valve between the stomach and intestines. When it swells shut, the condition is known as pyloric stenosis and causes infants to projectile vomit. It is uncommon, but when it occurs, it most often occurs in first-born males, usually around the first few weeks of life.

Self-full – most of the time we (especially women) are made to feel selfish when we do things for ourselves. A wise counselor once told me that when you do things for yourself, to take care of yourself, you are being selfFULL, not selfISH. In the spirit of "put on your oxygen mask first, and then help those around you," I have tried to be self-full. It empowers me to better help those I love.

The Global Hydranencephaly Foundation is a family driven nonprofit organization dedicated to providing families faced with a diagnosis of hydranencephaly the opportunity to help their child live the quality of life he or she deserves. The family-to-family resource network is the foundation of this mission: It is an ideally structured, multi-faceted community for the dissemination of invaluable information, sharing of effective care management strategies specific to the unique circumstances a family faced with a diagnosis of this rare neurological condition may encounter, and individualized, life-long support. Emphasis is placed on the development of empowered parent advocates, strengthened by the availability of comprehensive information, geographically tailored resources, and a confident awareness of the rights children have to quality, compassionate care without discrimination. We embrace the opportunity for continuous growth through the expansion of additional collaborative partnerships with like-minded organizations and reputable community businesses. Through community-based awareness campaigns and the planned infiltration of the medical community, we aim to conquer the misconceptions that exist surrounding this diagnosis and portray a clearer picture of the possibilities that exist for these children; giving multiple reasons to "Believe in the Impossible!" I am grateful to Global Hydranencephaly Foundation for allowing me to include their images.

Author Bio

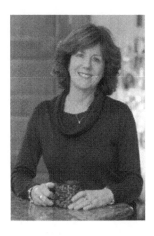

Theresa Jeevanjee teaches mathematics and computer science at Saint Louis University and for MEGSSS (Mathematics Education for Gifted Secondary School Students). She enjoys running, painting, cooking, and taking ballet classes. She is an associate in the CSJ (Congregation of St. Joseph) community and is active in three prayer groups. Her volunteer work includes tutoring mathematics, helping with the theatre and chorus costumes for her daughter's high school, and serving on the Collegium board (organization that supports faith and the intellectual life).

She and her husband live in Webster Groves, Missouri, with their children, Ryan, Kiran, and Lauren, and their two dogs, Ebony and Kuki.

To contact the author, please email faithandrelentlesslove@gmail.com.

For more information, please visit www.faithandrelentlesslove.com.

Printed in Great Britain
by Amazon.co.uk, Ltd.,
Marston Gate.